PROCEDURES SUPPLEMENT FOR

Introduction to Nursing

PROCEDURES SUPPLEMENT FOR

Introduction to Nursing

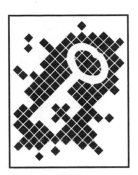

Barbara Kozier, BA, BSN, RN, MN

Glenora Erb, BSN, RN

Patricia McKay Bufalino, RN, MN

Addison-Wesley Publishing Company
Health Sciences
Redwood City, California · Menlo Park, California · Reading, Massachusetts
New York · Don Mills, Ontario · Wokingham, UK · Amsterdam · Bonn
Sydney · Singapore · Tokyo · Madrid · San Juan

Sponsoring Editor: Armando Parcés Enríquez

Production Coordinator: Brian Jones

Copy Editor: Wendy Earl

Text Designer: Gary Head

Cover Designer: Sue Gemmell

Illustrators: Jack P. Tandy, Sue Gemmell

Photographers: William Thompson, RN, Karen Stafford Rantzman, George Fry, Jeffry Collins, Marianne Gontarz, Mark Tuschman, David Barnett, Christopher Scott

The authors and publishers have exerted every effort to ensure that drug selections and dosages set forth in this text are in accord with current recommendations and practice at the time of publication. However, in view of ongoing research, changes in government regulations, and the constant flow of information relating to drug therapy and drug reactions, the reader is urged to check the package insert for each drug for any change in indications of dosage and for added warnings and precautions. This is particularly important where the recommended agent is a new and/or infrequently employed drug.

Addison-Wesley Publishing Company
Health Sciences
390 Bridge Parkway
Redwood City, California 94065

PREFACE

This *Procedures Supplement* was developed to give instructors a more complete range of procedures than could be included in *Introduction to Nursing*. Its 74 procedures, combined with the text's 62 procedures, offer all the skills that first-year nursing students need.

The chapter numbers in this *Procedures Supplement* coincide with the chapter numbers in *Introduction to Nursing*, but some chapters do not have any supplementary procedures. The contents pages list all the procedures presented in *Introduction to Nursing* as well as in this supplement. And each chapter in this supplement begins with a list of all the pro-

cedures in that chapter for both books. This *Procedures Supplement* does not repeat any procedure already presented in *Introduction to Nursing*.

This *Procedures Supplement* represents our continuing commitment and the commitment of the publisher to provide nurse educators with a variety of teaching materials in nursing fundamentals that can be adapted to fit almost any curriculum. We hope the students and instructors using *Introduction to Nursing* will find this supplement helpful and will continue to offer suggestions to improve its effectiveness.

Barbara Kozier

Glenora Erb

Patricia McKay Bufalino

DIRECTIONS
TO THE STUDENT

Specific nursing actions have been omitted from each procedure to avoid repetition. These actions, which underlie safe, competent nursing, are:

- Carry out a hand wash before gathering any clean or sterile supplies or before implementing a procedure, and after contact with a client, to avoid transmission of microorganisms to clients or to others.

- Implement appropriate blood and body fluid precautions (see inside front cover). The authors have suggested wearing gloves for most procedures that involve direct contact with any body fluid—although they do recognize that blood may not be present in the body fluid and that gloving may not always be necessary.

- Identify the client appropriately, eg, by reading the client's wrist band.

- Explain the procedure to the client and, in some instances, to support persons, adjusting your explanation to their needs. Explaining what you plan to do reassures people by letting them know what to expect. Explanations are provided in some procedures.

- Provide privacy for the client when any aspect of the procedure could be embarrassing to the client or to other people, and as an indication of respect for the client even when he or she is not conscious.

- Elevate the client's bed to a working level and lower the near side rail before starting a procedure. These actions help the nurse maintain good body mechanics.

- Following a procedure, lower the bed and raise the near side rail for clients requiring these precautions. These actions are taken for the client's safety.

- Ensure that the client is comfortable following the procedure.

- Dispose of used and unused supplies according to agency practice. This step includes cleaning and/or disinfecting equipment as necessary.

CONTENTS

PROCEDURES SUPPLEMENT FOR
Introduction to Nursing

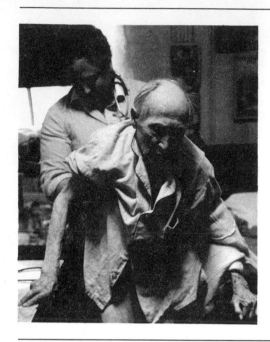

CHAPTER 4

HEALTH CARE DELIVERY SYSTEMS

■ New procedure:

Procedure 4–1
Admitting a Client to a Health Care Agency

> PROCEDURE 4–1   **Admitting a Client to a Health Care Agency**

Before admitting a client it is important to know the following:

1. The agency's policies and practices for admitting clients, in particular in regard to the client's medications, personal property, and security for valuables

2. The bed and/or room to which the client will be admitted

3. The client's general condition and/or medical diagnosis

4. Whether upon admission the client needs any special equipment such as an oxygen device

5. Whether the physician has written special orders to be implemented immediately upon the client's arrival

EQUIPMENT

- A stethoscope and a sphygmomanometer with a cuff to take blood pressure.

- A watch with a second hand to assess the client's pulse and respirations.

- A thermometer, if not provided at the bedside, to assess the client's temperature.

- A portable scale to assess the weight, in agencies that require this. In many agencies the client's weight and height are recorded as the client states them.

- A bedpan or urinal in which to acquire a specimen of urine if ordered.

- A urine specimen container and laboratory urinalysis requisition, both clearly labeled if a urine specimen is ordered.

- A hospital gown (and pajama bottoms for males) as necessary. Some agencies, or specific units, permit clients to wear their own night or lounge clothing or daytime dress. Psychiatric nursing units, for example, encourage full dress. Many medical-surgical nursing units, however, require clients to wear hospital gowns.

- A special envelope to enclose valuables for safekeeping if the admission office has not already provided one.

- A clothes list or clothing responsibility form. Some agencies have printed checklists of clothing and other personal effects that nurses can use to inventory the client's articles. A growing trend, however, is to place the clothes in a bedside locker and have the client sign a form assuming responsibility for them.

- Appropriate hospital forms, eg, a responsibility release for personal possessions.

- Labels to attach to the client's personal articles at the bedside, eg, a radio.

INTERVENTION

Preparing the Client's Room

After notification by the nurse in charge that a new client will be admitted to the nursing unit, the nurse assigned prepares the client's room for the arrival.

1. Open a closed bed for the client's convenience.

2. In most cases, place the bed in a low position or place a footstool by a bed that is not adjustable, to make it easier and safer for the client to get into bed. If you know that the client is being transported by stretcher, however, place the bed in a high position to facilitate transfer from stretcher to bed.

3. Check that all necessary unit supplies are provided: a full water jug if not contraindicated, a bedpan or urinal, a bath basin, a kidney basin, a call signal, etc.

4. Provide equipment essential to the client's specific needs. Such equipment could include an intravenous pole, a footboard, an overhead frame with a trapeze, and oxygen equipment.

Meeting the Client

5. Greet the client in a manner that conveys interest and concern. Call the client by the name he or she desires, introduce yourself, and inquire about any immediate problems that the client may have. If the client is feeling distraught or upset, take time to listen and talk, to allay these concerns. If the client is in acute pain, attend to this at once, contacting the physician for medication orders and/or providing other nursing interventions.

Rationale By attending to the client's immediate problems, the nurse indicates a primary concern for the client's welfare. This makes the client feel that problems will be attended to, and it does much to initiate a sense of security and a trusting relationship.

6. Obtain other essential information about the client's physical and emotional status from the client's record or health team members.

Rationale This assists the nurse in attending to the client's immediate problems.

Preparing the Client

7. Explain what the admission entails and how the client can participate.

Rationale Although the admission procedure often becomes routine for health personnel, it is unfamiliar to clients.

8. Provide privacy when the client undresses and when he or she gives a urine specimen.

9. Direct support persons to the lounge area unless they can assist the client to undress. Reassure them that they will be called when it is best for them to return. On pediatric units the admission procedure is often carried out in the treatment room with the active participation of the support person.

Orienting the Client to the Unit

10. Introduce the client to the other clients in the room and to any staff members encountered, even though the client cannot be expected to remember all their names. Tell the client the name of the nurse in charge of the unit and that person's role.

Rationale Introduction to roommates facilitates the client's adjustment to the agency; introduction to staff members helps the client recognize caregivers. Knowing the name of the nurse in charge and her or his problem-solving role helps the client feel more secure and provides a means for the client to communicate problems.

11. Explain and demonstrate use of equipment.
    a. Explain how the call system works.
    b. Explain equipment in the bedside table and location of his or her locker.
    c. Show location of the bathroom and showers.
    d. Demonstrate overhead room lighting and night lighting.

e. If applicable, demonstrate use of a bedside television.

Rationale Knowledge about location and appropriate use of equipment ensures the client's safety.

12. Provide information about the agency to the client and support persons.
    a. Inform the client about meal hours and nourishment times.
    b. Explain visiting hours and policies.
    c. Describe other areas in the hospital that the client or support persons may use, such as lounges, the cafeteria, the chapel, and the canteen.
    d. Explain how the client may obtain a television or radio.
    e. Inform the client of smoking regulations.
    f. Describe facilities and services available, such as gift shop, library, newspaper delivery, cafeteria, chapel, and chaplain visitation.
    g. Inform the client of the location of the public telephone and operation of the portable or bedside telephone.

    Rationale Knowledge of the agency's policies promotes the client's and support person's feelings of security and minimizes anxiety. Many agencies provide information pamphlets that cover most of this information. Check what materials are available in your agency.

13. Describe the staff's expectations of the client. For example, tell the client what to wear, to remain in his or her room until the doctor has visited, or to inform the nursing staff of his or her whereabouts.

Admitting the Client

14. Assist the client to change into hospital gown or, if agency policy allows, personal sleeping garments. Many clients do not require assistance undressing but need to be informed which way to put on a hospital gown, ie, with the ties at the back.

    Rationale Because the physical examination is an essential part of the admission procedure, the client's body parts are more readily exposed if a gown or pajamas are worn.

15. Assist the client as needed to a comfortable position in bed or in a chair.

Rationale Client comfort reduces anxiety and tension, which can elevate cardiac and respiratory rates and blood pressure. Accuracy of assessment findings is essential for baseline data used to compare subsequent findings.

16. Place the clothes in the bedside locker and either list the clothes or have the client sign a form assuming responsibility for them, following the policy of the agency. Some agencies have support persons take the client's clothing home.

17. Inform the client of agency policy about valuables. Special envelopes are usually provided by the agency to store valuables such as money, jewelry, and keys in a locked safe in the business office. Supply an envelope, if this is agency policy. Assure the client that the valuables will be safely handled and returned at discharge. Have the client sign a statement absolving the hospital of responsibility for valuables kept at the bedside. Agency policies generally state the amount of money the client should keep at the bedside. Clients undergoing prolonged hospitalization sign special release forms to be able to withdraw small amounts of money from safekeeping as needs arise. Label large items, such as radios, with the client's full name.

18. Provide a container for dentures if the client requires one and discuss precautions about storing them.

    Rationale A proper storage place for dentures reduces the chance of damage to them.

19. Ask whether the client has brought medications. If so, request that they be taken home or send them to the hospital pharmacy or designated area for safekeeping. It is usual for only certain medications, such as nitroglycerin, to be kept at the bedside. Check agency policy.

    Rationale While the client is in the hospital, medications must be carefully regulated to be therapeutic and to avoid incompatibilities.

20. Take the client's temperature, pulse, respirations, blood pressure, height, and weight. In some agencies the blood pressure is not taken for children under 6, however.

    Rationale These vital signs provide baseline data for subsequent assessments during hospitalization. They are indicators of the client's general condition.

21. Obtain a urine specimen if ordered. Explain to the client the reason for it, eg, to detect an infection of the urinary tract. Direct ambulatory clients to the bathroom to provide a specimen. Provide a bedpan or urinal for bed clients to use. Apply a urine collector to children who are not toilet-trained.

    Rationale A urine specimen is ordered if there is a reason to suspect a urinary problem. Because it is not cost effective, urinalysis is no longer a routine screening procedure in many agencies.

22. Obtain a nursing assessment. (See Procedure 8–1.)

    Rationale The nursing assessment provides baseline data for subsequent care planning.

23. Inform the client that a blood specimen and chest x-ray film will be taken by a technician, if applicable.

    Rationale A blood specimen is routinely taken from many or all clients, to do a hemoglobin assessment, blood typing, and crossmatching for clients having surgery. Some agencies are also doing routine AIDS screening. Chest x-ray films may be taken to ascertain the presence of any lung disease such as tuberculosis.

24. Inform the client of any treatment to be administered in the near future, eg, during the next shift or day. For example, clients who are having surgery need to know what preoperative preparations (such as surgical shave) are required.

    Rationale Knowledge of what to expect reduces anxiety.

25. Place the call signal within easy reach of the client, ensure that the bed is in the low position and that side rails are raised if indicated.

26. Inform support persons when they can return, and inform them about visiting hours.

    Rationale Consideration of support persons conveys your understanding of their concern and needs.

27. Send specimens to the laboratory with appropriate labels and requisitions.

28. Place allergy alerts, if necessary, on the client and the chart, according to agency policy. Record allergies in red ink, both on the front of the client's chart and on the nursing Kardex. A sign indicating specific allergies may also be placed on the foot of the client's bed or on the wall above the head of the bed. If the client has food allergies, notify the dietary department.

    Rationale Allergy alerts prevent constant questioning of the client when therapies are administered, serve as reminders to caregivers, and safeguard the client.

29. Record assessment data on the appropriate forms of the client's record, in accordance with agency procedure. For example, some agencies record the vital signs on both the nurse's notes and the graphic record. Selected data from the nursing assessment form are generally transferred to the nurse's notes as well as the client's Kardex. Record on the nurse's notes and on the valuables envelope the disposition of the valuables.

Sample Recording

Date	Time	Notes
12/5/89	11:40	Admitted walking. T 97, P 82, R 14, BP on "L" arm 130/70. Is alert. States is in to have gallbladder removed, has no discomfort at present. States has no known allergies. States takes thyroid pills twice a day before breakfast and at bedtime. Clean voided urine specimen sent to lab. Gave watch and ring to wife to take home. $50.00 cash placed in valuables envelope and given to hospital Business Office to place in safe. Oriented to hospital routines and equipment. Given information pamphlet about preop prep. ——————————————Sheila S. Murphy, NS
	11:50	Dr. L. Stein notified of admission. ——————————Sheila S. Murphy, NS
	12:30	Blood sample for CBC, Hb, blood typing and cross-matching taken by lab technician. ——Sheila S. Murphy, NS

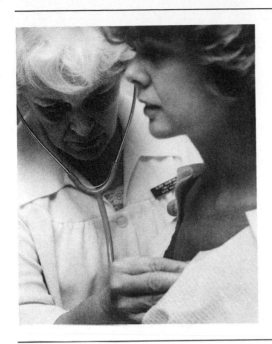

CHAPTER 8

ASSESSING

■ New procedure:

Procedure 8–1
Performing a Nursing Assessment

PROCEDURE 8–1 **Performing a Nursing Assessment**

Careful assessment is a crucial aspect of the admission procedure, since incomplete or inaccurate assessment can lead the nurse to make incorrect nursing diagnoses, resulting in inappropriate client goals and intervention. A nursing assessment is a systematic method of collecting desired data about the client. When performing a nursing assessment, the nurse follows a systematic framework.

There are many frameworks for a nursing assessment. Theories, models, frameworks, and principles are all used as approaches for the data collection. Some nursing models provide an assessment tool to help the nurse gather data.

The nurse's interviewing skills are extremely important during a nursing assessment. Because problem identification and clarification is an integral part of this process, this interview is exploratory in nature. Interviewing principles and guidelines must be followed to elicit desired information and to set a therapeutic tone for the nurse-client relationship.

EQUIPMENT

- A nursing assessment form if available.

INTERVENTION

1. Observe the client's general appearance.

   Rationale Objective data used in conjunction with the subjective data provided by the client enables the nurse to formulate accurate nursing diagnoses.

2. Determine the client's current health status and health history as follows:

   a. Ask the client his or her reason for admission to the agency. Focus on the client's own perception or views for entering the agency. Ask about the client's chief discomforts and complaints, and have the client comment about those things that are most problematic. Use the client's own words when possible when recording data.

   Rationale Focusing on the client's views assists the nurse to assess the client's knowledge about and causative factors of the problem. Comments about the most problematic concerns help to set priorities. Listening to and documenting the client's own words assists in identifying acuity of distress and discomfort.

   b. Obtain the client's history of illnesses and where and why he or she was previously hospitalized. Include the physician's name if known.

   Rationale Knowledge of past illnesses may indicate relationship to current illness and lifestyle patterns.

   c. Determine which medications have been taken routinely or recently and their doses and frequency. If the client is unable to provide the names of the medications, list them by their actions (eg, water pill, BP pill, heart pill, etc). Determine the method used to administer medications (eg, in liquid or pill form).

   d. Ensure that the assessment lists all allergies to food, medications, and substances that may cause contact dermatitis (soaps, creams, lotions, and ointments). If allergies are not known, write "not known" or "none known."

   Rationale To ensure safe and appropriate therapy for the client, it is essential that all allergies are documented and that allergy bands are provided.

   e. Acquire data about frequency of substance use. Include use of tobacco; use of alcohol, coffee, tea, and other caffeinated drinks such as colas; use of sleeping or mood-altering medications; and use of mind-altering drugs such as marijuana. Explain the reason for such data. Some clients may feel more comfortable providing this data when other family members are not present.

   Rationale Data about substance use and abuse provides information about the client's life-style, possible factors contributing to illness, and the client's coping patterns. Being sensitive to the client's need for privacy and giving a reason for such data helps the nurse obtain information that is relatively accurate and not distorted due to embarrassment.

3. Obtain data about the client's methods and abilities to manage the activities of daily living (ADL).

   Rationale Data about the client's ADL provide the nurse with clues about life-style or risk factors that may contribute to potential or actual health problems and about assistance required with self-care.

   a. *Eating patterns:* Ask whether the client is on a special (eg, low-salt, low-fat, or kosher) diet.

Document the client's usual eating patterns and food preferences.

b. *Sleep/rest patterns:* Inquire about difficulties with sleeping and any aids used to facilitate sleep (eg, glass of milk at bedtime, medications). Have the client also describe rest and relaxation patterns.

c. *Elimination patterns:* Ask if the client has any problems with urinary and fecal elimination. If problems exist, ask how the client manages them. For example, does the client use fecal-elimination aids such as laxatives?

d. *Activity/exercise patterns:* Have the client describe his or her pattern of exercise, activity, leisure, and recreation. Determine whether the client has activity and mobility limitations such as limited joint range of motion that affect dressing or walking.

e. *Use of prostheses:* Inquire about the specific type of prostheses the client uses, eg, upper, lower, or partial dentures; eyeglasses or contact lenses; hearing aids; wig; mastectomy or limb prostheses; colostomy, ileostomy, or ureterostomy appliances. When appropriate, determine how the client manages each prosthesis and whether there are problems associated with management of it. For example, what is the condition of the skin around a colostomy? How often does the client clean his or her contact lenses or hearing aid?

4. Obtain specific social and family data about the client.

a. *Languages spoken:* Determine whether English is or is not spoken and understood and what other languages are spoken. For clients who do speak English, determine whether English is their primary or first language. Document the fact that English is a second language or is not spoken and what specific languages are spoken and understood.

Rationale This data may indicate the need for an interpreter or the fact that the client, if able, may be used as an interpreter.

b. *Occupation or school:* Assess the type of work and current employment status of adults and how they feel their illness will affect their employment. For children determine their current school status (ie, grade), whether special classes are attended, and their attitude toward school.

Rationale Serious employment concerns can indicate the need for support and counseling; long-term illnesses in children may indicate the need for a home instructor.

c. *Family/home situation:* List family members by age and determine what major health problems other family members have. Have the client describe his or her perception of how the illness or hospitalization affects family members. Ask which family members or friends will be visiting the client.

Rationale Knowledge of the family situation and friends provides the nurse with data about support systems for the client and possible stresses on the family unit and client.

d. *Religious practices:* Ask the client what religious practices he or she routinely performs and how these can be supported throughout the illness.

Rationale Continuance of religious practices provides spiritual support for the client.

e. *Financial status:* Ask the client about any financial concerns in regard to health care.

Rationale Financial status may influence the client's decisions regarding health care.

5. Document all pertinent assessment findings on the client's record and complete the assessment record with your signature.

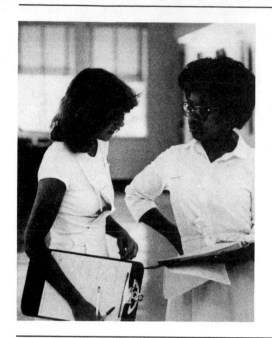

RECORDING AND REPORTING

■ New procedures:

Procedure 22–1
Transferring a Client

Procedure 22–2
Discharging a Client

PROCEDURE 22–1 **Transferring a Client**

Clients may be transferred (moved) to another unit within the agency, to another bed within the unit, or to another agency. Some transfers are required because of the client's health or undertaken at the client's request. Examples of reasons for transferring are

- To obtain special care, eg, in an intensive care unit

- To obtain a different type of accommodation, such as a single room rather than a four-bed room

CLIENT'S BELONGINGS AND SUPPLIES

- All the client's personal belongings, eg, clothes in locker, slippers, clothes in drawers, dentures, cosmetics, magazines, books. Place the belongings in the client's suitcase or in bags provided by the agency.

- The equipment used at the bedside, eg, bedpan, urinal, washbasin, towels, emesis basin, denture cup. Some agencies leave this equipment at the bedside and provide another set at the new bed. Check agency policy.

- The client's record and related supplies, such as medication cards, the nursing care plan, medications. Write a discharge summary as required.

INTERVENTION

Nurse in Current Unit

1. Assess the client's current health status as appropriate; eg, note respirations, blood pressure, pulse, condition of skin.

2. Explain to the client about the transfer. Be sure to explain that the hospital's information desk will be given the new room number so that visitors can be told.
   Rationale Many clients worry about change and are reassured by knowing the reason for the transfer, what the other nursing unit is like, when the move will take place, and any arrangements that are being made.

3. Establish the method by which the client can move, such as by wheelchair or stretcher. This may be indicated in the client's record or by the nurse. Clients normally are transferred by wheelchair unless they are too ill to sit up.

4. Lock the wheels on the stretcher or wheelchair when the client moves on and off it.
   Rationale Locking prevents the wheels from moving and thus endangering the client's safety.

5. Assist the client to the wheelchair or stretcher. Provide warm coverings as needed.
   Rationale Assistance prevents undue exertion. Coverings prevent chilling and maintain the client's sense of modesty.

6. Record in the chart the time of the transfer, the unit to which the client is moving, the mode of transport—eg, by wheelchair—and any significant assessments including the condition of the client. This recording is completed just prior to moving the client (see the sample recording following the procedure).

7. Take the client and the supplies to the other unit, or arrange for transport service.

8. Stop at the nurses' station upon arrival at the receiving unit, and introduce the nurse in charge to the client. Review the client's record or discharge summary with a nursing staff member (receiving nurse) on the new unit.

9. Leave the chart, medications, and nursing care plan at the nurses' station.

10. Take the client to the new room and assist him or her into bed. The receiving nurse should go with you. Ensure that the client is comfortable.

11. Return to your nursing unit with the stretcher or wheelchair.

12. Notify the information desk and other departments (such as the dietary department and pharmacy) of the transfer. Most agencies have a list of the departments that need to be notified when a client is transferred. Often this is done in writing.

13. At the client's former bed unit, strip the bed and arrange for *terminal cleaning*. In some agencies, housekeeping personnel carry out this cleaning; in others, nursing personnel do it.

Nurse in Receiving Unit

14. With the transferring nurse, review the client's chart or discharge summary (if written) and the assessments, nursing diagnoses, etc. This is par-

ticularly important when interventions are carried out just prior to the transfer, eg, administration of an analgesic.

15. Assess the client's immediate health and provide any interventions immediately needed. Record data in the client's record.

16. Welcome the client and any accompanying support persons. Introduce other clients in the room. Orient the client to any practices that are different on this unit from those of the previous unit.

17. Confirm that other departments, such as the dietary department, know the new location of the client.

18. Record on the client's chart the time of arrival, method of transport, and assessment data.

Sample Recording: Transferring Nurse

Date	Time	Notes
6/12/89	11:00	Transferred by wheelchair to A6. P 96, BP 160/90. All personal items, including dentures, moved with client. Meds given to L. Jones, RN ——————————Eliza L. Begbie, NS

Sample Recording: Receiving Nurse

Date	Time	Notes
6/12/89	11:15	Received by wheelchair. Color pale. P 106, BP 160/90. C/o fatigue. Oriented to unit practices. Dr. Bedow notified. ——————————Karen S. Stockley, NS

PROCEDURE 22–2 **Discharging a Client**

When clients leave a hospital, they are normally discharged with the physician's authorization (a written order by the physician—eg, "May go home tomorrow"—on the client's chart).

Usually, clients plan and look forward to their discharge from the hospital. Several health professionals—such as a dietitian, a social worker, and a community health nurse—may be working with the hospital nurse, client, and support persons to make discharge plans.

EQUIPMENT

- Any equipment the client requires, eg, walker, crutches, oxygen source.

INTERVENTION

Before Day of Discharge

1. Collaborate with the client, significant others, and/ or the home care nurse regarding needs required in the home.

   Rationale   Adaptations in the home environment can often contribute to independent functioning and to a client's safety.

2. Establish a teaching program for the client and significant others as soon as convenient during hospitalization. The program could teach how to give injections, colostomy care, diet. Provide written information when possible.

   Rationale   People usually need time to practice new skills and ask questions. Written information can be referred to after discharge.

3. Provide the client and/or significant other with information about community health resources that may be helpful.

   Rationale   Most communities have a variety of services that can support the client and help meet his or her health needs, eg, meals-on-wheels, day-care centers for the elderly.

4. Complete a referral form. See Figure 22–1.

Day of Discharge

1. Arrange to discuss health care with the client and/or significant others.

   Rationale   They may have last-minute questions.

2. Determine whether and at what time the client has made arrangements for transportation. At many hospitals if an ambulance is required, the nurse telephones to make the arrangements.

   Rationale   Usually, clients and/or support persons are responsible for making arrangements for their own transportation.

3. If there are valuables in safekeeping, obtain the client's signature on the release form and return the valuables.

4. Confirm that the business office has completed its procedures. If it has not, make arrangements for the client to visit the office or for an office representative to visit the client. Arrangements for paying are usually made at the time of admission.

5. Determine if there are any medications or prescriptions for the client.

6. Assess the client's health status, eg, inspect the surgical dressing, assess the pulse and blood pressure.

7. Contact the transport service or obtain a wheelchair if required for the client, unless an ambulance will be used. Obtain a utility cart to transport personal effects if the client cannot hold them.

   Rationale   Because of the danger of overexertion, some hospitals require that a wheelchair be used even though the client feels able to walk. The ambulance crew will have a stretcher for the person who needs an ambulance.

8. Lock the wheels of the chair. Raise the foot supports. Then assist the client into the wheelchair and support the feet appropriately.

   Rationale   Locking the wheels prevents the chair from moving and endangering the client's safety.

9. Take the client and the personal effects to meet the arranged transportation.

10. Lock the wheels of the chair and raise the foot supports before assisting the client to move.

11. Assist the client to the transportation and place the personal effects inside it.

12. Report to the nurse in charge and/or the unit clerk that the client has been discharged.

Patient Name: *Mr. Donald Phillips*

Medical Record Number: *5447652001*

INTER-AGENCY REFERRAL FORM
ALLIED HEALTH INFORMATION

Address Reply To:
STANFORD UNIVERSITY HOSPITAL
Patient Care Planning Program
300 Pasteur Drive
Stanford, CA 94305-5232

(addressograph stamp)

Medicare No. *0721569702*	Medi-Cal No.	From (Ward or Clinic) *4 SOUTH*	(415) 725- *4499*

Admission Date: *7/15/89*	Discharge Date: *8/1/89*	Medications Administered Day of Discharge:

Name and Address of Nearest ~~Relative or~~ Friend:
KAY JONES (neighbor)
14 MONTGOMERY ST., MENLO PARK, CA

Medications Administered Day of Discharge:
COUMADIN 5mg @ 0900 hrs.

NURSING EVALUATION

	GOOD	FAIR	POOR
Vision	✓		
Hearing		✓	
Speech			✓
Bladder Control			✓
Bowel Control		✓	
Date of last BM	*7/31/89*		

PATIENT USES:	YES	NO	COMMENTS
Glasses	✓		
Hearing Aide	✓		
Dentures	✓		
Catheter *(Condom)*	✓		Type: △'d:
Tubes		✓	Type: △'d:
Prosthesis		✓	Type:
Colostomy		✓	△'d:

	MOBILITY		PERSONAL NEEDS	
	Walks		Call Bell	
	Cane	A	Feeds Self	
	Crutches		Eating Device	
	Walker	A	Commode	
A	Wheelchair		Bedpan	
A	Bed/Chair	I	Urinal	
	Bedfast	A	Bathing	
		I	Wash Face	
		A	Shave/Make-Up	
		I	Comb Hair	
		A	Brush Teeth/Dentures	

CODE:
I = Independent
A = Assist
D = Dependent

PATIENT IS:	YES	Describe Atypical Behavior
Alert/Appropriate		
Confused		
Combative		
Noisy		
Withdrawn	✓	*DEPRESSED ABOUT DYSPHASIA*
Wanderer		

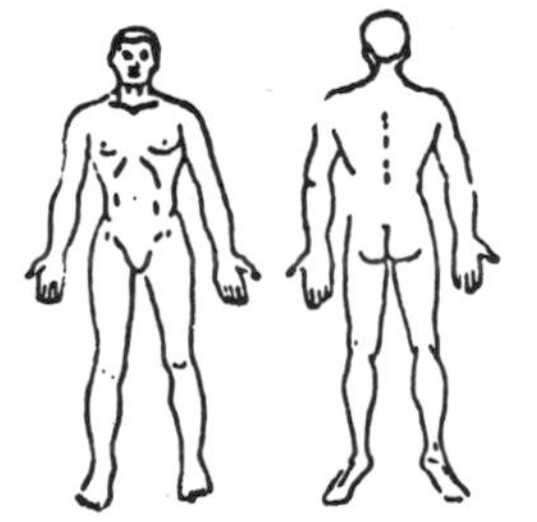

SKIN (describe), DRESSING CHANGES, or TREATMENTS:
SKIN DRY BUT INTACT. SLING APPLIED TO (L) ARM

Myra Brown RN 7/31/89
SIGNATURE — TITLE — DATE

PHYSICAL AND OCCUPATIONAL THERAPY:
ROM exercises to (L) arm and (L) leg daily. Quadriceps exercises to (R) leg. *Larry Agnew, PT 7/31/89*
SIGNATURE — TITLE — DATE

DIET: *No RESTRICTIONS*

TEACHING:
SIGNATURE — TITLE — DATE

SOCIAL (Current/future living arrangements; family composition, etc.)
AND OTHER PERTINENT INFORMATION:
THIS 86 YR. OLD WIDOWER LIVES ALONE. HAS ONE DAUGHTER (IN NEW YORK CITY) WHO IS EXPLORING LONG TERM CARE FACILITIES IN THIS AREA. CLIENT'S ATTEMPTS TO VERBALIZE NEED TO BE ENCOURAGED. HE UNDERSTANDS SLOW, DISTINCT SPEECH. *Myra Brown RN 7/31/89*
SIGNATURE — TITLE — DATE

REPLY TO BE COMPLETED WITHIN 4 WEEKS:

SIGNATURE — TITLE — DATE

Figure 22–1
An inter-agency referral form. SOURCE: From Stanford University Hospital, Stanford, California. Reprinted with permission.

EL CAMINO HOSPITAL

LEAVING HOSPITAL AGAINST ADVICE

Date...

This is to certify that..
a patient in the above named hospital, is leaving the hospital against the advice of the attending physician and the hospital administration. I acknowledge that I have been informed of the risk involved and hereby release the attending physician, and the hospital, from all responsibility and any ill effects which may result from this action.

....
Patient

....
Other Person Responsible

....
Relationship

Witness...

Witness...

Figure 22−2
A discharge form for a client who is being released against medical authority.
SOURCE: El Camino Hospital, Mountain View, California. Reprinted with permission.

13. Document on the client's chart the discharge, the time, the method of transport to the agency door, and assessment data. Some agencies also suggest that the client's destination, eg, a nursing home, be included in the discharge notes.

Sample Recording

Date	Time	Notes
12/5/89	1400	Discharged by wheelchair to Sunnyvale Lodge. Meds taken by wife. Written instructions provided about leg exercises. ———Maria L. Chevez, NS

14. Write a discharge profile if this was not done before the client left the unit.

15. Determine that the record for discharge has been completed. If not, leave it in the appropriate place for the physician. Once it is completed, send the record to the records office.

16. Return to the client's room and arrange for terminal cleaning of the unit.

Considerations for the Elderly

Discharge planning must consider any existing age-related disabilities, eg, reduced visual acuity, decreased strength, impaired memory. Special aids, such as seven-day pill dispenser, can be used to help clients keep track of their medications. Also, discharge planning must include support for ADL. Often there are special agencies in the community to assist elderly clients following discharge from a hospital.

Discharging a Client AMA

Occasionally, clients leave an agency without the permission of the physician. These are *unauthorized discharges*, often referred to as discharge against medical authority (AMA), and the client is asked to sign a special form releasing the hospital from any responsibility after the departure. See the sample release in Figure 22−2.

It is important the person understand that refusing a particular treatment or medication is not the same as refusing all treatments and desiring to leave the hospital. The AMA form is used in the latter instance, whereas refusing a particular aspect of care is the client's right and needs to be documented on the chart and reported to the nurse in charge.

When a client decides to leave a health care facility AMA, the following activities are indicated:

1. Ascertain why the person wants to leave the agency.

   Rationale Sometimes clients have misunderstood information or have fears the nurse can resolve. As a result, the client may be desirous of staying in the agency.

2. Notify the physician.

3. Offer the client the appropriate form to complete (see Figure 22–2).

4. If the client refuses to sign the form, document the fact on the form and have another health professional witness this.

5. Provide the client with the original of the signed form and place a copy in his or her record.

6. When the client leaves the agency, notify the physician, nurse in charge, and agency admimistration as appropriate.

7. Assist the client to leave as if this were a usual discharge from the agency.

   Rationale The agency is still responsible while the client is on the premises.

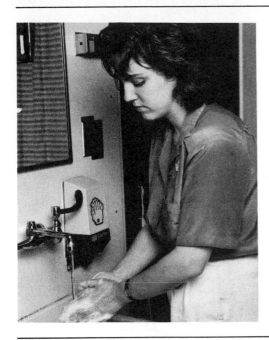

CHAPTER **23**

PREVENTING THE TRANSFER OF MICROORGANISMS

☐ The following procedures appear in *Introduction to Nursing:*

Procedure 23–1
Handwashing

Procedure 23–2
Establishing and Maintaining a Sterile Field

Procedure 23–3
Donning and Removing Sterile Gloves (Open Method)

■ New procedure:

Procedure 23–4
Donning a Sterile Gown and Sterile Gloves (Closed Method)

PROCEDURE 23–4 **Donning a Sterile Gown and Sterile Gloves (Closed Method)**

Sterile gowning and closed gloving are chiefly carried out in the operating room or delivery room. Prior to these techniques, the nurse dons a hair cover and a mask.

EQUIPMENT

- A sterile pack containing a sterile gown and sterile gloves. In some agencies the gloves are provided in a separate package.

INTERVENTION

Donning a Sterile Gown

1. Open the sterile pack.

2. Remove the outer wrap from the sterile gloves, and drop the gloves in their inner sterile wrap on the sterile field established by the sterile outer wrapper. By not touching the inner wrapper, it remains sterile. See Procedure 23–2 in *Introduction to Nursing.*

3. Carry out a surgical scrub for the length of time required by the agency. See Procedure 46–6.

4. Grasp the sterile gown at the crease near the neck, hold it away from you and permit it to unfold freely without touching anything, including your uniform.

   Rationale The gown will be unsterile if its outer surface touches any unsterile articles.

5. Put your hands inside the shoulders of the gown and work your arms partway into the sleeves without touching the outside of the gown. See Figure 23–1.

6. If donning sterile gloves by using the closed method (see steps 8–16 below), work your hands down the sleeves only to the proximal edge of the cuff.

   or

   If donning sterile gloves by using the open method, work your hands down the sleeves and through the cuffs.

7. A coworker wearing a hair cover and mask grasps the neck ties without touching the outside of the gown and pulls the gown upward to cover the

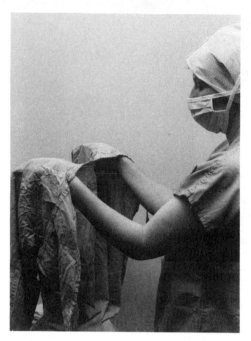

Figure 23–1

neckline of your uniform in front and back. The coworker ties the neck ties. Gowning continues at step 17.

Donning Sterile Gloves (Closed Method)

8. While the hands are still covered by the sleeves, open the inner sterile wrapper containing the sterile gloves. See Figure 23–2.

9. With your dominant hand, pick up the opposite glove with your thumb and index finger, handling it through the sleeve.

10. Lay the glove on the opposite gown cuff, thumb side down, with the glove opening pointed toward the fingers. See Figure 23–3. Position your nondominant hand palm upward inside the sleeve.

11. With the nondominant hand, grasp the cuff of the glove through the gown cuff and firmly anchor it.

12. With your dominant hand working through its sleeve, grasp the upper side of the glove's cuff and stretch it over the cuff of the gown.

13. Pull the sleeve up to draw the cuff over the wrist

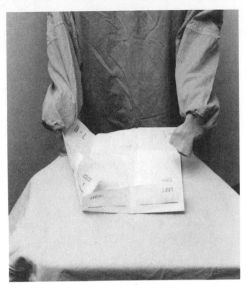

Figure 23–2

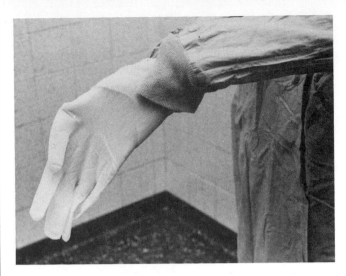

Figure 23–4

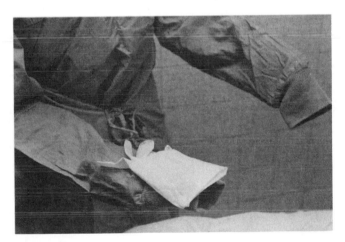

Figure 23–3

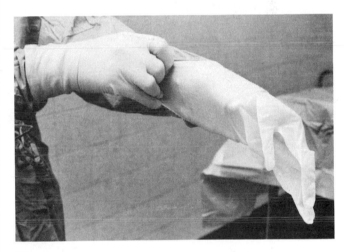

Figure 23–5

as you extend the fingers of the nondominant hand into the glove's fingers. See Figure 23–4.

14. To don the second glove, place the fingers of the gloved hand under the cuff of the remaining glove.

15. Place the glove over the cuff of the second sleeve.

16. Extend the fingers into the glove as you pull the glove up over the cuff. See Figure 23–5.

Completion of Gowning

17. A coworker who is masked and whose hair is covered holds the waist tie of your gown, using sterile gloves or a sterile wrapper or drape.

Rationale   The tie remains sterile.

18. Make a three-quarter turn, then take the tie, and secure it in front of the gown.

 or

A coworker wearing sterile gloves takes the two ties at each side of the gown and ties them at the back of the gown, making sure that your uniform is completely covered.

Rationale   In both methods the back of the gown remains sterile.

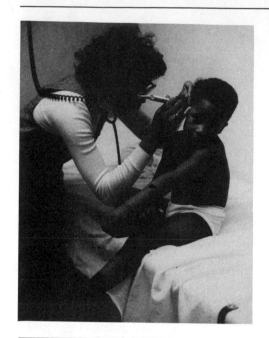

ASSESSING HEALTH STATUS

Because assessment is an integral part of the nursing process, aspects of specific assessment techniques should be used in all nursing interventions. The assessment required by an individual at a given time is a nursing judgment based upon knowledge and the client's health needs.

PROCEDURE 32–4 **Measuring the Height of a Child or Adult**

Height is measured starting at the age when children can stand. It is measured in centimeters or in feet and inches, depending on the agency's practice.

Height and weight measurements are extremely important in assessing the growth of infants and children. Height is an essential measurement, along with weight, to determine safe dosages of medications to give to infants and children.

EQUIPMENT

- A measuring stick. Some weight scales have a built-in measuring stick. There are also measuring sticks that can be placed against or attached to a wall.

- (Optional) A paper protector on which the bare-footed client stands, to prevent the spread of microorganisms.

- A ruler, book, or measuring square.

INTERVENTION

1. Make sure the client is able to stand independently or with assistance.

2. Assist the client to the appropriate place for measurement, and help him or her to remove shoes or slippers. If the client will be barefooted after removing shoes or slippers, place a paper protector on the platform of the scale.

3. Assist the client to stand on the scale with his or her back against the measuring stick. The client stands erectly with heels together; with heels, buttocks, and occiput (back of the head) against the measuring stick; and with eyes looking straight ahead.

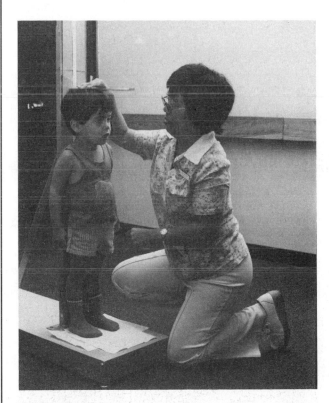

Figure 32–1

Rationale An erect posture ensures a correct measurement.

4. Place the ruler, book, or measuring square on top of the client's head at a right angle to the measuring stick. See Figure 32–1.

5. Determine the point on the measuring stick to which the bottom side of the ruler or book comes.

6. Assist the client to put on shoes or slippers and to resume activity or assume a comfortable position in bed.

7. Discard the protector, if used, in the waste container.

   Rationale The protector will possess microorganisms from the client that could be transmitted to others.

8. Assess the midpoint of the stature (optional). For the newborn it is approximately at the umbilicus; for the adult it is at the symphysis pubis.

9. Determine the ratio of sitting height to total body height (optional). This decreases with age until the extremities stop growing. In the newborn, sitting height is about 70% of body length; in the 3-year-old, about 57%; in girls at the time of menarche and in boys at age 15, about 52%. The sitting height then increases a few percentage points, since the trunk continues to grow slightly after the extremities have completed growth.

10. Document the client's height in the appropriate place. Heights are often recorded on the graphic sheet.

PROCEDURE 32–5   **Measuring the Weight of a Child or Adult**

Weight is often measured on a client's admission to a health agency. The weight of some clients is measured regularly, eg, each morning before breakfast. This regular weighing is usually done for obese clients on reducing diets or for clients who retain excess fluid (edema).

Weight is measured in kilograms or pounds. A person who weighs 100 lb is calculated to weigh 45.45 kg, as follows.

$$2.2 \, lb = 1 \, kg$$

$$100 \, lb \times \frac{1 \, kg}{2.2 \, lb} = \frac{100 \, kg}{2.2} = 45.45 \, kg$$

A person who weighs 80 kg is calculated to weigh 176 lb, as follows.

$$2.2 \, lb = 1 \, kg$$

$$80 \, kg \times \frac{2.2 \, lb}{1 \, kg} = 176 \, lb$$

EQUIPMENT

- A suitable scale.
- A protector for the scale. For a standing scale use a clean paper towel on which the barefooted client can stand. When a canvas sling or chair is used, it should be protected by a plastic cover that can be readily cleaned after use.

INTERVENTION

1. Place the scale next to the client's bed or assist the client to the location of the scale.

2. Lock the wheels of the scale to prevent it from slipping.

3. Provide privacy as necessary. Clients do not usually undress, but, if repeated (eg, daily) weighings are done, the client should wear the same amount of clothing each time and the measurement should be taken on the same scale at the same time of day. In a hospital, clients usually wear their hospital gowns or pajamas. Clients usually remove shoes or slippers before being weighed.

4. If the client will be barefooted, place a paper protector on the platform of a standing scale.

Rationale   The protector prevents the transfer of microorganisms from the scale to the feet.

5. Check that the scale registers 0. Adjust it, if necessary.

For a Standing Scale

6. Assist the client onto the scale. Make sure the client is not leaning on the bed or holding a chair. If the client is unsteady, remain nearby to assist. Be sure the client stands on the center of the platform.

   Rationale   Standing in the center is necessary both for accurate measurement and for safety.

7. Read the weight on the dial or adjust the counterbalance to obtain the weight. Determine whether the scale is in pounds or kilograms.

8. Assist the client off the scale. Dispose of the paper protector, if used, in the waste container.

9. Document the weight on the client's chart.

For a Bed Scale

10. Check the manufacturer's instructions.

11. Adjust the scale stretcher to a horizontal position and lock it in place.

12. Turn the client to a lateral position, with his or her back toward the scale.

13. Roll the base of the scale under the bed; widen the base (if adjustable).

    Rationale   The wider base provides maximum stability.

14. Lock the wheels.

15. Lower the stretcher onto the bed so that it is centered on the bed.

16. Roll the client onto the stretcher.

17. Move the weighing arms over the client and attach them securely to the stretcher.

18. Gradually pump the handle to raise the client 5 cm (2 in.) above the bed surface. Pump slowly and evenly to avoid jerking the client.

19. Ensure that the stretcher is not touching any part of the bed or its attachments.

Rationale Touching any equipment will affect the reading of the weight.

20. Press the button (on a digital scale) to display the weight. Adjust the counterbalance on a balance scale or refer to the dial on a dial scale.

21. After observing the weight registered, lower the client gradually to the bed by using the pump handle.

22. Detach the stretcher from the arms.

23. Roll the client off the stretcher.

24. Remove the stretcher, and assist the client to a comfortable position.

25. Release the lock on the wheels. Clean the scale and return it to storage with the stretcher in the vertical position.

26. Record the weight on the client's chart.

For a Chair Scale

27. Check the manufacturer's instructions.

28. Position the chair scale beside the client, and lock the wheels.

29. If the side arm nearest the client moves, unlock it, and move it away from the chair.

    Rationale This can facilitate the client's transfer.

30. Transfer the client onto the chair of the scale. Transferring a client between a bed and a chair is discussed in Procedure 36–12.

31. Return the arm, and lock it in place.

    Rationale The arm provides additional security.

32. Adjust the counterbalances or read the digital display.

33. Unlock the chair arm, and transfer the client back to the bed or a wheelchair.

34. Unlock the wheels, lock the balance arm, clean the scale, and return it to storage.

    Rationale An unlocked balance arm can be damaged during movement.

35. Record the weight on the client's chart.

CHAPTER **33**

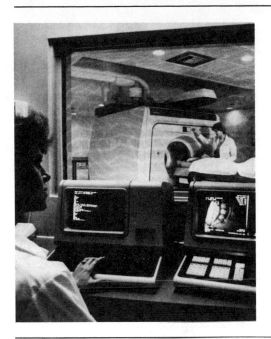

ASSISTING WITH SPECIAL PROCEDURES

■ New procedures:

Procedure 33–1
Assisting with a Lumbar Puncture

Procedure 33–2
Assisting with an Abdominal Paracentesis

PROCEDURE 33–1 **Assisting with a Lumbar Puncture**

In a lumbar puncture (LP, or spinal tap) cerebrospinal fluid (CSF) is withdrawn by inserting a needle into the subarachnoid space of the spinal canal, between the third and fourth lumbar vertebrae or between the fourth and fifth lumbar vertebrae. At this level the needle avoids damaging the spinal cord and major nerve roots. See Figure 33–1. An LP is carried out by a physician. Strict sterile technique is essential to prevent the introduction of microorganisms into the spinal canal. Lumbar punctures are carried out for a variety of reasons:

- To analyze the constituents of a specimen of fluid for diagnostic purposes

- To test the pressure of the CSF for diagnostic purposes

- To relieve pressure by removing CSF

- To inject a spinal anesthetic, dye, or air into the spinal canal

- To inject a medication, ie, intrathecal chemotherapy

The physician locates the appropriate intervertebral space, disinfects the site, drapes the area with sterile drapes, and administers a local anesthetic. After the area is numbed, the physician inserts the spinal needle with the stylet and removes the stylet. When the flow of CSF is ascertained, the stopcock and manometer are attached, and an initial CSF pressure reading is taken at the point where the CSF stops rising in the manometer tube. Normal opening pressures are 60–180 mm of water. Pressures above 200 mm are considered abnormal.

A Queckenstedt-Stookey test may also be done while the manometer is in place. The nurse may be asked to exert digital (finger) pressure on one or both of the internal jugular veins. See Figure 33–2. The normal response is an increase in CSF pressure.

The physician usually takes specimens of CSF and hands the specimen tubes to the nurse, who numbers them in the sequence taken. A total of 10 mL of fluid is generally collected, with 2–3 mL of fluid in each specimen tube. Specimens of CSF are often tested in the laboratory for the presence of certain elements (eg, protein, sugar, bacteria) and cell count.

After collecting the specimens, the physician may take a final, or closing, CSF pressure reading before removing the spinal needle.

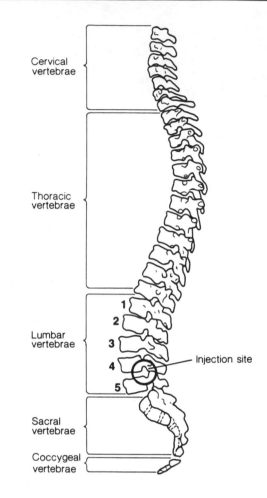

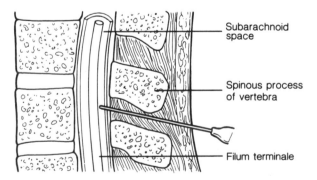

Figure 33–1
A diagram of the vertebral column, indicating a site for insertion of the lumbar puncture needle into the subarachnoid space of the spinal canal.

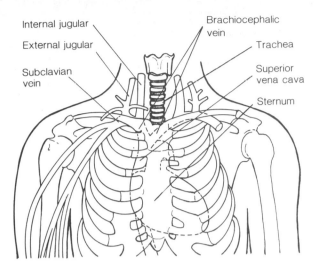

Figure 33–2
Location of the internal jugular vein for the
Queckenstedt-Stookey test.

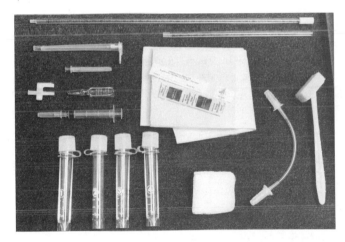

Figure 33–3
A preassembled lumbar puncture set. Note the
manometer at the top of the set.

EQUIPMENT

- A sterile lumbar puncture set. See Figure 33–3.
  The set contains:
  - Sterile sponges or gauze squares with an antiseptic solution to apply to the site of the puncture.
    If the skin antiseptic is not included in the set, a
    container of it must be obtained.
  - Drapes. One may be *fenestrated.*
  - A syringe and needle to administer the local anesthetic. A 2-mL syringe and #24 and #22 needles
    are often provided.

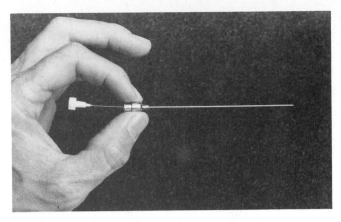

Figure 33–4
A spinal needle with the stylet protruding from the hub.

- A spinal needle 5–12.5 cm (2–5 in.) long, with
  a stylet to insert into the spinal canal. See Figure
  33–4. The shorter needle is used for infants.
- A manometer (a glass or plastic tube calibrated in
  millimeters) to measure the pressure of CSF.
- A three-way stopcock (a valve between the spinal
  needle and the manometer that regulates the flow
  of CSF by shutting off the CSF drainage, allowing
  the CSF to flow either into the manometer or out
  into a receptacle).
- Specimen containers (test tubes).
- A local anesthetic, eg, 1% procaine, to anesthetize the lumbar site. This may or may not be
  included in the preassembled set. If included, it
  will be supplied in a small glass ampule. If not
  included, a vial or ampule must be obtained.
- A small dressing to apply over the puncture site.
- Face masks (optional).
- Sterile gloves.
- A completed laboratory requisition and specimen
  labels.
- Gloves to protect the nurse from contact with cerebrospinal fluid.

INTERVENTION

Preprocedure

1. Obtain assessment data.
2. Explain the following:
   a. That the physician will be taking a small sample of spinal fluid from the lower spine.

b. That a local anesthetic will be given so that the client will feel little pain.

c. When and where the procedure will occur, eg, at the bedside or in the treatment room.

d. Who will be present, ie, the physician and the nurse.

e. The time involved, eg, about 15 minutes.

In addition, tell the client what to expect during the procedure. The client may feel slight discomfort (like a pinprick) when the local anesthetic is injected and a sensation of pressure when the spinal needle is being inserted. Remind the client that it is important to remain still and in one position throughout the procedure. A restless client or a child will need to be held to prevent movement.

3. Have the client empty his or her bladder and bowels prior to the procedure to prevent unnecessary discomfort.

4. Position the client laterally with the head bent toward the chest, the knees flexed onto the abdomen, and the back at the edge of the bed or examining table. See Figure 33–5. Place a very small pillow under the client's head to maintain the horizontal alignment of the spine. In this position the back is arched, increasing the spaces between the vertebrae so that the spinal needle can be inserted readily.

5. Drape the client to expose only the lumbar spine.

6. Open the lumbar puncture set, and supply the physician with the sterile gloves and antiseptic. The physician may want the antiseptic in the container or poured onto the sterile gauze squares.

During the Procedure

7. Stand in front of the client, and support the back of the neck and knees if help is required to remain still. See Figure 33–5. Reassure the client throughout the procedure by explaining what is happening. Encourage the client to breathe normally and to relax as much as possible.

   Rationale Excessive muscle tension, coughing, or changes in breathing can increase CSF pressure, giving a false reading.

8. If the Queckenstedt-Stookey test is being done, place digital pressure on the client's jugular veins. See Figure 33–2.

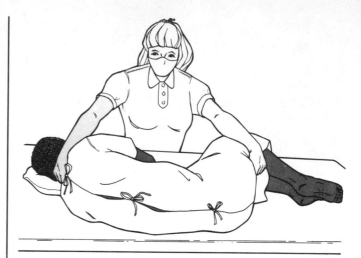

Figure 33–5

9. Label the specimen tubes in sequence if they are not already labeled. While handling the tubes, take care to prevent contamination of the physician's sterile gloves, the sterile field, and yourself, since the CSF may contain virulent microorganisms, eg, organisms that cause meningitis. Don gloves before handling test tubes because the outside may have been in contact with the CSF.

10. Observe the client's color, respirations, and pulse during the lumbar procedure.

11. Place a small sterile dressing over the site of the puncture to help prevent infection after the needle is removed.

Postprocedure

12. Assist the client to a dorsal recumbent position with only one head pillow. The client remains lying down for 8–24 hours, until the spinal fluid is replaced. Determine the recommended time this position should be maintained. Some clients experience a headache following a lumbar puncture, and the dorsal recumbent position tends to prevent or alleviate it. Often analgesics are ordered and can be given for headaches.

13. Assess the client's response to the procedure, eg, pallor; feeling of faintness; changes in pulse rate and other vital signs; changes in neurological status; headache; swelling or bleeding at the puncture site; and numbness, tingling, or pain radiating down the legs, which may be due to nerve

irritation. Report any unusual reactions to the nurse in charge.

14. Ensure that the CSF specimens are correctly labeled and immediately send them with the completed requisition to the laboratory. CSF specimens are normally not refrigerated.

15. Document the procedure on the client's chart, including the date and time it was performed; the name of the physician; the color, character (clear, cloudy, etc), and amount of CSF obtained; the pressure readings; the number of specimens obtained; and the nurse's assessments and interventions.

Sample Recording

Date	Time	Notes
5/24/89	1500	Lumbar puncture performed by Dr Guido. Four 2 mL specimens of cloudy serous CSF sent to lab. Initial pressure 130 mm. Closing pressure 100 mm. No apparent discomfort. Resting. —Sarah D. Nicols, NS

16. Regularly assess for headache, take vital signs, and assess neurologic status.

PROCEDURE 33–2 **Assisting with an Abdominal Paracentesis**

Normally, the peritoneum creates just enough peritoneal fluid for lubrication. The fluid is continuously formed and absorbed into the lymphatic system. However, in some disease processes, a large amount of fluid accumulates in the cavity; this condition is called *ascites*. Normal ascitic fluid is serous, clear, and light yellow. An abdominal paracentesis is carried out to obtain a fluid specimen for laboratory study and to relieve pressure on the abdominal organs due to the presence of excess fluid.

The procedure is carried out by a physician with the assistance of a nurse. Strict sterile technique is followed. A common site for abdominal paracentesis is midway between the umbilicus and the symphysis pubis on the midline. See Figure 33–6. The physician disinfects the site of the incision, drapes the area with sterile drapes, and administers a local anesthetic. After the area is numbed, the physician makes a small incision with a scalpel, inserts the trocar and cannula (the trocar inside the cannula), and then withdraws the trocar. Tubing is attached to the cannula and the fluid flows through the tubing into a receptacle. Normally, about 1500 mL is the maximum amount of fluid drained at one time, to avoid hypovolemic shock. The fluid is drained very slowly for the same reason. Some fluid is placed in the specimen container before the cannula is withdrawn. The small incision may or may not be sutured; in either case, it is covered with a small sterile bandage.

EQUIPMENT

- A sterile set containing:
  - Sterile sponges or gauze squares with an antiseptic solution.
  - A drape (or drapes) to place over the client's abdomen. The drape is often fenestrated, and the opening is placed at the site where the fluid will be removed.
  - A 2-mL syringe and #24 and #22 needles to administer the anesthetic.
  - A small scalpel to make an incision in the abdomen. A needle holder and sutures to sew up the incision after withdrawing the fluid.
  - A receptacle for the fluid.
  - An aspirating set. The *trocar* is a sharp pointed instrument that fits inside the *cannula*. The cannula is a tube through which plastic tubing can

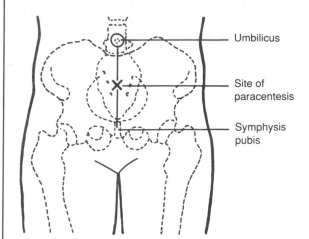

Figure 33–6
A common site for an abdominal paracentesis.

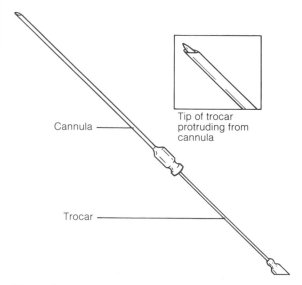

Figure 33–7
A trocar and cannula may be used for an abdominal paracentesis.

be threaded to drain the fluid. See Figure 33–7. If the purpose of the paracentesis is to obtain a specimen, the physician may use a long aspirating needle attached to a syringe rather than making an incision and using a trocar and cannula.

- Specimen containers.
- A local anesthetic.

- Masks (optional).

- Sterile gloves for the physician.

- Nonsterile disposable gloves for the nurse.

- A completed laboratory requisition and a label for the specimen.

INTERVENTION

Preprocedure

1. Obtain assessment data.

2. Weigh the client.

3. Measure the abdominal girth at the level of the umbilicus. Often the level is marked so that the same level is used when measuring the girth postprocedure. See Figure 33–8.

   Rationale   To obtain an indication of the amount of ascites.

4. Explain the procedure to the client. Normally, an abdominal paracentesis is not painful, and, when a client has considerable ascites, the procedure can relieve discomfort caused by the fluid. The procedure to remove ascitic fluid usually takes 30–60 minutes. Obtaining a specimen usually takes about 15 minutes. Emphasize the importance of remaining still during the procedure. Include in your explanation when and where the procedure will occur and who will be present.

5. Have the client void just before the paracentesis to lessen the possibility of puncturing the urinary bladder. Notify the physician if the client cannot void.

6. Help the client assume a sitting position in bed so that the fluid accumulates in the lower abdominal cavity, and the force of gravity and the pressure of the abdominal organs will help the flow of the fluid from the cavity. Some clients may be able to sit on the edge of the bed with pillows to support the back. Cover the client to expose only the necessary area.

During the Procedure

7. Open the paracentesis set, and supply the physician with the sterile gloves. Supply the antiseptic from the container or pour it onto sterile gauze squares. Don disposable nonsterile gloves.

8. Open and hold the ampule or vial of local anesthetic if it is not part of the sterile set.

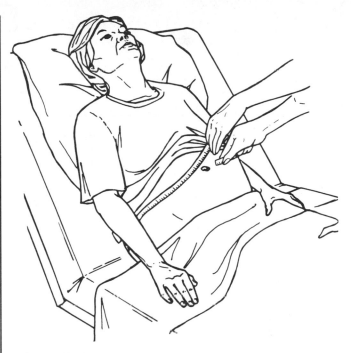

Figure 33–8

9. Support the client verbally, and describe the steps of the procedure if the physician does not do so.

10. Observe the client closely for signs of distress. A major concern is hypovolemic shock induced by the loss of fluid. See step 12.

11. Place a small sterile dressing over the site of the incision after the cannula or aspirating needle is withdrawn.

Postprocedure

12. Assess the client's response in terms of pulse rate, skin color, and blood pressure. Hypovolemic shock can occur when the fluid in the circulatory system is redirected to the abdominal area as a result of reduced pressure from the removal of the ascitic fluid. Shock is evidenced by pallor, dyspnea, diaphoresis (profuse perspiration), and a drop in blood pressure.

13. Measure the abdominal girth with a tape measure in the same place as before the procedure.

14. Arrange for the specimen with the completed requisition and label to be transported to the laboratory.

15. Record the procedure on the client's chart, including the date and time; the name of the physician; the girth of the client's abdomen before and after the procedure; the color, clarity, and

amount of drained fluid; and any nursing assessments and interventions.

Sample Recording

Date	Time	Notes
7/18/89	1400	Paracentesis performed by Dr Johnson, 300 mL clear serosanguinous fluid obtained. Abdominal girth at umbilical level 114 cm before, 109 cm after. Specimen sent to laboratory. P 72, BP 120/85. Slight pallor. Resting comfortably. ———————Roxanne J. Tuttle, NS

16. Regularly assess for hypovolemic shock, signs of infection (elevated body temperature), and signs of internal hemorrhage (lowered blood pressure; accelerated pulse; hard, boardlike abdomen).

CHAPTER 34

PERSONAL HYGIENE

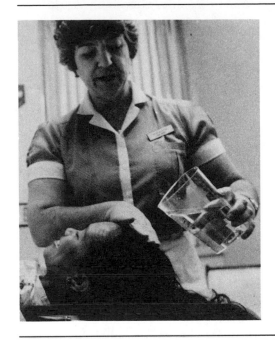

☐ The following procedures appear in *Introduction to Nursing:*

Procedure 34–1
Bathing an Adult

Procedure 34–2
Perineal-Genital Care

Procedure 34–3
Giving a Back Rub

Procedure 34–4
Providing Special Oral Care

Procedure 34–5
Changing an Unoccupied Bed

■ New procedures:

Procedure 34–6
Changing a Hospital Gown for a Client with an Intravenous Infusion

Procedure 34–7
Shaving a Male Client

Procedure 34–8
Foot Care

Procedure 34–9
Cleaning Artificial Dentures

Procedure 34–10
Shampooing Hair (Client Confined to Bed)

Procedure 34–11
Removing Contact Lenses (Hard and Soft)

Procedure 34–12
Cleaning Contact Lenses (Hard and Soft)

Procedure 34–13
Inserting Contact Lenses (Hard and Soft)

Procedure 34–14
Removing, Cleaning, and Inserting a Hearing Aid

Procedure 34–15
Changing an Occupied Bed

Hygiene practices involve care of the skin, hair, nails, teeth, oral and nasal cavities, eyes, ears, and, in women, the vagina. Although hygiene practices are generally done independently and personally, the very young, the elderly, and the physically and mentally ill often require assistance from a nurse. Attending to hygienic needs not only increases the client's feeling of self-worth but also is effective in maintaining the health of the integument and preventing infection.

PROCEDURE 34–6   **Changing a Hospital Gown for a Client with an Intravenous Infusion**

A client may require a gown change while an intravenous (IV) infusion is running into the arm. Some hospitals provide special gowns for clients receiving IVs. These gowns open from the neck over the shoulders and down the sleeves. The openings are closed with ties or Velcro fasteners that can be undone on the side with the IV, so that the sleeve slips readily off the client when the gown needs to be removed. Another practice is to remove the gown sleeve from the client's arm before an IV is started. Again, this makes it simple to change the gown.

EQUIPMENT

- A clean hospital gown
- Clean bed linen, if required
- A basin of water, soap, a washcloth, and a towel, if needed for washing the client

INTERVENTION

1. Inspect the intravenous site and the arm.

2. Count the rate of flow of the infusion.
   Rationale   It should be running at the designated rate.

Removing a Soiled Gown

3. Remove the gown from the arm without the infusion.
   Rationale   It is easier to remove the sleeve from the arm with the infusion last.

4. Slip the gown down the arm with the IV and onto the tubing. See Figure 34–1.

5. Take the intravenous container off the hook and slide the sleeve over it. See Figure 34–2. Maintain the position the container was in when hanging, and hold it above the client's arm. Do not pull on the tubing.
   Rationale   Maintaining the container's position prevents the backflow of blood from the vein into the tubing. Pulling on the tubing can dislodge the needle in the vein.

6. Remove the soiled gown. Rehang the intravenous container. Wash and dry the client as necessary.

Putting a Clean Gown on the Client

7. Put the gown in front of the client as it would be worn.

8. Take the intravenous container off the hook, and pass it through the sleeve from the inside to the cuff. See Figure 34–3. Maintain the position the container was in on the stand, and keep it above the level of the arm.

9. Rehang the intravenous container.

10. Carefully guide the client's arm and the tubing into the sleeve. Be careful not to pull on the tubing.

11. Arrange the tubing so that it is gently coiled. Avoid any kinks.
    Rationale   Kinks can stop the flow of the solution into the client's vein.

12. Assist the client to put the other arm into the second sleeve of the gown.

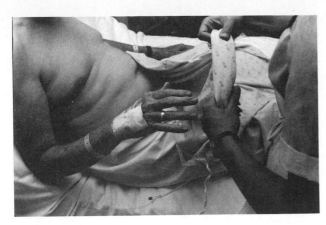

Figure 34-1

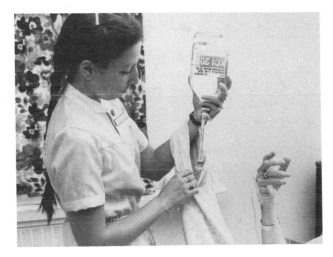

Figure 34-2

13. Secure the ties on the gown at the back of the neck.

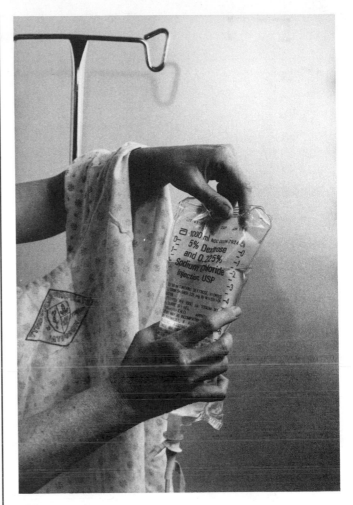

Figure 34-3

14. Count the rate of flow of the infusion to make sure it is correct.

PROCEDURE 34–7 **Shaving a Male Client**

A man who is accustomed to being clean shaven may feel unkempt and ashamed of his appearance when whiskers grow on his face. Moreover, after 2–3 days of whisker growth, the skin of the face can become irritated.

EQUIPMENT

- A razor and sharp blade or an electric razor. Most people have their own equipment and have a preference.

- Shaving cream or shaving soap and a shaving brush. The client may have a preference.

- A bath towel, a face towel, and a washcloth. These protect the bed and the client from moisture and are used for wiping and drying the face.

- A bath blanket to cover the chest. This maintains warmth and keeps the client dry.

- A basin with hot water at 46 C (115 F) or the temperature the person prefers.

- After-shave lotion or powder, according to the client's preference.

- A mirror.

INTERVENTION

1. Assess the facial skin for reddened, bruised, or broken areas.

2. Determine the amount of assistance the client requires and whether the agency permits nurses to shave male clients. Some hospitals provide barbers and do not permit nurses to shave male clients except in special circumstances, eg, when the client is on protective aseptic precautions. Also determine whether a physician's order is required before shaving.

3. Assist the client to a sitting position or to as convenient a position as possible for him.

4. Fold the bedclothes to the waist if the client is remaining in bed, and place a bath blanket around his shoulders if he feels chilly.

5. If the client is in bed, place a towel under his head to protect the pillow from moisture.

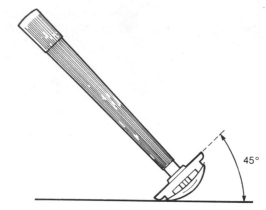

Figure 34–4

6. Starting on one side of the face, lather the cheek from below the sideburn to the jaw. Hot water and shaving soap usually provide a good lather. Do not apply soap if you will be using an electric razor.

   Rationale Hot water and shaving soap soften the beard bristles for easier removal and decrease skin irritation from the razor blade.

7. Hold the razor so that the blade is at a 45° angle to the skin. See Figure 34–4.

   Rationale This angle decreases the chances of nicking the skin.

   or

   With an electric razor, start on one side, and work in the direction the hair grows (downward), making short strokes. Empty the razor when it becomes full of hair. Stretch the skin tautly to shave in creases.

8. Shave in the direction of the hair (downward), using short, firm strokes about 2.5 cm (1 in.) long.

   Rationale Longer strokes are more likely to pull the hairs.

9. Dip the razor in hot water to remove the lather and hair after each downward set of strokes.

   Rationale These materials can clog the razor and prevent effective cutting.

10. Apply lather and shave the following areas:
    a. The second cheek.
    b. The upper lip.
    c. The chin.

Pull the skin taut with the other hand before shaving areas with creases, such as the chin.

Rationale Keeping the skin taut helps prevent cutting the skin.

11. Wipe the face with a wet washcloth to remove any remaining shaving cream and hair.

12. Dry the face well with the face towel.

13. Inspect the face for any unshaven areas and cuts. Assist the client to inspect the shave in the mirror. If an area was missed, lather and shave it.

14. Apply after-shave lotion or powder (as the man prefers) to the shaved area of the face, using a patting motion with the fingers.

Rationale Rubbing can irritate the skin.

15. Document assessments, such as extreme fatigue, and any facial skin problems. Shaving is not normally recorded.

PROCEDURE 34–8 **Foot Care**

Foot care is of particular importance when the client has an infection or abrasion, diabetes mellitus, or impaired circulation to the extremities. The latter two conditions predispose people to infections. These individuals need to learn proper foot care to prevent problems. Other clients normally care for their own feet. After determining a person's personal foot care practices, the nurse can identify the learning needs. Foot care is usually provided in conjunction with the bed bath but can be provided at any time.

EQUIPMENT

- A washbasin
- Thermometer to test the water temperature
- Soap
- A washcloth
- Towels
- A moisture-resistant disposable pad
- Lotion
- Toenail cleaning and trimming equipment

INTERVENTION

1. Assess the feet for any lesions, reddened, dried or cracked areas.

2. Fill the washbasin with 40.5 C (105 F) water.
   Rationale Warm water promotes circulation, is comforting, and is refreshing.

3. Assist the ambulatory client to a sitting position in a chair; assist the person confined to bed to a supine or semi-Fowler's position as health permits.

4. Place a pillow under the knees of the person in bed.
   Rationale The pillow provides support and prevents muscle fatigue.

5. Place the washbasin on the moisture-resistant pad at the foot of the bed or, for an ambulatory client, on the floor in front of the chair.

6. Pad the rim of the washbasin with a towel for the person in bed.

Rationale The towel prevents undue pressure on the skin.

7. Place one foot in the basin.

8. Allow the client's foot to soak for at least 10 minutes. Rewarm the water as needed.
   Rationale Soaking softens the skin and nails and loosens debris under the toenails.

9. Wash the foot with soap, and rinse it. Rub callused areas of the foot with the washcloth.
   Rationale Friction created by rubbing removes dead skin layers.

10. Remove the foot from the basin and place it on the towel.

11. Blot the foot gently with the towel to dry it thoroughly, particularly between the toes.
    Rationale Harsh rubbing can damage the skin and cause thrombosis. Thorough drying reduces the risk of infection.

12. Apply lotion.
    Rationale Lotion moistens dry skin.

13. Observe the foot for any problems.

14. Empty the washbasin, refill it with water, and soak and clean the other foot.

15. While the second foot is soaking, clean and trim the toenails of the first foot, if permitted. In many agencies toenail trimming is contraindicated for clients with toe infections or peripheral vascular disease, unless performed by a podiatrist or physician.

16. Repeat trimming for the second foot.

17. Document all assessments. Foot care is not generally recorded unless problems are noted.

Considerations for the Elderly

Elderly people who have poor circulation should avoid colored hosiery because the dye can sometimes irritate the skin. Also, avoid constricting items such as tight knee-high hosiery, which can decrease circulation further.

PROCEDURE 34–9 **Cleaning Artificial Dentures**

Some people have artificial teeth in the form of a plate—a complete set of teeth for one jaw. A person may have a lower plate and/or an upper plate. When only a few artificial teeth are needed, the individual may have a bridge rather than a plate. Artificial teeth are fitted to the individual and usually will not fit another person.

Most people prefer privacy when they take their artificial teeth out to clean them. Many do not like to be seen without their teeth; one of the first requests of postoperative clients is often, "May I have my teeth in, please?"

Like natural teeth, artificial dentures collect microorganisms and food. They need to be cleaned regularly, at least once a day. They can be removed from the mouth, scrubbed with a toothbrush, rinsed, and reinserted. Some people use a dentifrice, while others use commercial cleaning compounds for plates.

EQUIPMENT

- A denture container, such as a small basin or plastic cup, in which to carry the dentures.
- A toothbrush or stiff-bristled brush to scrub the dentures.
- A dentifrice or denture cleaner.
- Tepid water to wash and rinse the dentures.
- A clean washcloth to place in the sink.
- A container of mouthwash.
- A curved basin, such as a kidney basin, to receive the mouthwash after rinsing.
- A towel to wipe hands and mouth.
- A tissue or piece of gauze to obtain a secure hold to remove the dentures (optional).
- Gloves to protect the nurse.

INTERVENTION

1. Assist the client to a sitting or side-lying position so that it is easier to spit out mouthwash without swallowing it.
2. Don gloves.

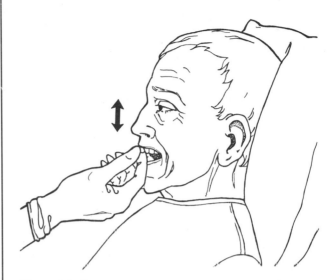

Figure 34–5

To Remove Dentures

3. If the client cannot remove the dentures, grasp the upper plate at the front teeth with your thumb and second finger, and move the denture up and down slightly. See Figure 34–5.

   Rationale The slight movement breaks the suction that holds the plate on the roof of the mouth.

4. Lower the upper plate, move it out of the mouth, and place it in the denture container.

5. Lift the lower plate, turning it so that the left side, for example, is slightly lower than the right, to remove the plate from the mouth without stretching the lips. Place the lower plate in the denture container.

6. Remove a partial denture by exerting equal pressure on the border of each side of the denture, not on the clasps, which can bend or break.

7. To clean dentures, take the denture container to a sink. Take care not to drop the dentures because they may break. Place a washcloth in the bowl of the sink.

   Rationale A washcloth prevents damage to the dentures if the nurse drops them.

8. Using a toothbrush or special stiff-bristled brush, scrub the dentures with the cleaning agent and tepid water.

Rationale Hot water is not used because heat will change the shape of some dentures.

9. Rinse the dentures with tepid running water.

   Rationale Rinsing removes the cleaning agent and food particles.

10. If the dentures are stained, soak them in a commercial cleaner. Be sure to follow the manufacturer's directions. To prevent corrosion, dentures with metal parts should not be soaked overnight. Home substitutes for commercial cleaner are the following mixtures:

    a. 5–10 mL (1–2 tsp) white vinegar and 240 mL (1 cup) warm water.

       or

    b. 5 mL (1 tsp) chlorine bleach, 10 mL (2 tsp) water softener, and 240 mL (1 cup) warm water. It is essential to mix water softener with the bleach to prevent denture corrosion and to rinse well before replacing in the mouth.

11. Observe the dentures for any rough, sharp, or worn areas that could irritate the tongue or mucous membranes of the mouth, lips, and gums.

12. Inspect the mouth for any redness, irritated areas, or indications of infection.

13. Return the dentures. Before inserting them, offer some mouthwash and a curved basin to rinse the mouth. If the client cannot insert the dentures independently, insert the plates one at a time. Hold each plate at a slight angle while inserting it, to avoid injuring the lips. See Figure 34–6.

14. Assess the fit of the dentures.

15. Assist the client to wipe hands and mouth with the towel.

16. If the client does not want to or cannot wear the dentures, store them in a denture container with water. Label the cup with the client's name and identification number.

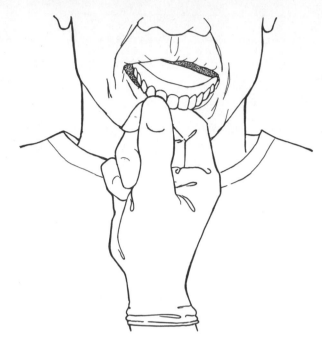

Figure 34–6

17. Remove gloves and discard.

18. Document all assessments and include any problems, such as an irritated area on the mucous membranes of the mouth. Report problems to the nurse in charge. Cleaning dentures is not normally recorded. The location of dentures if not worn is recorded.

Considerations for the Elderly

Elderly people who have dentures should see a dentist at least once a year to check the fit, occlusion, and the presence of any irritation to the soft tissues of the mouth. Elderly clients who need repairs to their dentures or new dentures may need a referral for financial assistance to correct problems.

PROCEDURE 34-10   **Shampooing Hair (Client Confined to Bed)**

The frequency of shampooing the hair varies considerably among individuals. Many people wash their hair weekly; some shampoo less often than weekly; and a number shampoo daily.

Clients who are ill may shampoo hair by several methods, depending on their health, strength, and age. The client who is well enough to take a shower can conveniently shampoo while in the shower. The client who is unable to shower may be given a shampoo while sitting on a chair in front of a sink. The back-lying client who can move to a stretcher can be given a shampoo on a stretcher wheeled to a sink. The person who must remain in bed can be given a shampoo with water brought to the bedside. The latter is the least convenient method.

EQUIPMENT

- A comb and a brush.

- A shampoo basin to catch the water and direct it to the washbasin or other receptacle. Shampoo basins are usually made of plastic or metal. If one is not available, a plastic drawsheet can be rolled up on three sides to make edges about 7 cm (3 in.) high. These edges will guide the water to the receptacle, in which the unrolled fourth edge of the sheet is placed.

- A receptacle for the shampoo water. A pail or a large washbasin can be used. If possible, the receptacle should be large enough to hold all the shampoo water so that it does not have to be emptied during the shampoo.

- A pitcher of water. The water should be 40.5 C (105 F) for an adult or child to be comfortable and not injure the scalp.

- A bath thermometer to measure the temperature of the water.

- Two bath towels.

- A plastic sheet or pad to protect the bedclothes.

- A bath blanket to cover the upper part of the client for warmth.

- A washcloth or pad to support the client's neck.

- A liquid or cream shampoo. Usually, the person will supply this. If the shampoo is being given to destroy lice, the physician will order the shampoo to be used.

- A conditioner to facilitate combing the wet hair.

- A hair dryer.

INTERVENTION

1. Assess the hair and scalp.

2. Determine whether a physician's order is needed before a shampoo can be given. Some hospitals require an order.

3. Determine the type of shampoo to be used, eg, a medicated shampoo.

4. Determine the best time of day for the shampoo. Discuss this with the client. A person who must remain in bed may find the shampoo tiring. Choose a time when the client is rested and can rest after the procedure.

5. Assist the client to the side of the bed from which you will work.

6. Remove pins and ribbons from the hair, and brush and comb it to remove any tangles.

7. Put the plastic sheet or pad on the bed under the head.
   Rationale   The plastic keeps the bedding dry.

8. Remove the pillow from under the client's head, and place it under the shoulders.
   Rationale   This hyperextends the neck.

9. Tuck a bath towel around the client's shoulders.
   Rationale   The towel keeps the shoulders dry.

10. Place the shampoo basin under the head, putting a folded washcloth or pad where the client's neck rests on the edge of the basin. If the client is on a stretcher, the neck can rest on the edge of the sink with the washcloth as padding.
    Rationale Padding supports the muscles of the neck and prevents undue strain and discomfort.

11. Fanfold the top bedding down to the waist, and cover the upper part of the client with the bath blanket.
    Rationale   The folded bedding will stay dry, and the bath blanket, which can be discarded after the shampoo, will keep the client warm.

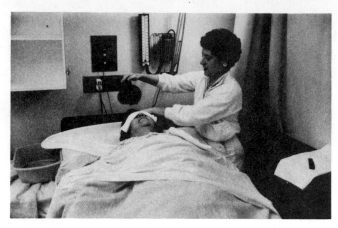

Figure 34-7

12. Place the receiving receptacle on a table or chair at the bedside. Put the spout of the shampoo basin over the receptacle.

13. Place a damp washcloth over the client's eyes. See Figure 34-7.

    Rationale The washcloth protects the eyes from soapy water. A damp washcloth will not slip.

14. Place cotton fluffs in the client's ears if indicated.

    Rationale These keep water from collecting in the ear canals.

15. Wet the hair thoroughly with the water.

16. Apply shampoo to the scalp. Make a good lather with the shampoo while massaging the scalp with the pads of your fingertips. Massage all areas of the scalp systematically, eg, starting at the front and working toward the back of the head.

    Rationale Massaging stimulates the blood circulation in the scalp. The pads of the fingers are used so that the fingernails will not scratch the scalp.

17. Rinse the hair briefly, and apply shampoo again.

18. Make a good lather and massage the scalp as before.

19. Rinse the hair thoroughly this time to remove all the shampoo.

    Rationale Shampoo remaining in the hair may dry and irritate the hair and scalp.

20. Squeeze as much water as possible out of the hair with your hands.

21. Rub the client's hair with a heavy towel.

22. Remove the shampoo equipment from the bed, and assist the person confined to bed to a comfortable position.

23. Dry the hair with the dryer. Set the temperature at "warm" and continually move the dryer to prevent burning the client's scalp.

24. Arrange the hair using a clean brush and comb.

25. Document the shampoo and any assessments. Report problems noted to the nurse in charge.

Sample Recording

Date	Time	Notes
6/2/89	1300	Shampoo given. Abrasion 2.5 cm long on right occipital area. Area appears pink with some bluish discoloration surrounding it. White scaly area on left temporal area 4 cm in diameter. Dr King notified.————— Kim L. Krueger, SN

≈ Considerations for the Elderly

Because body oils decrease with age, the hair tends to become drier and more brittle. Shampooing hair should be no more often than once a week to keep it clean. Frequent brushing increases the blood supply to the scalp and increases the flow of natural oils.

PROCEDURE 34–11   **Removing Contact Lenses (Hard and Soft)**

Contact lenses, thin curved discs of hard or soft plastic, fit on the cornea of the eye directly over the pupil, to correct visual defects. They float on the tear layer of the eye. Contact lenses may also be gas permeable.

Most clients normally care for their own contact lenses. There are a number of ways to place contact lenses on the eyes and to remove them. People learn the method that best suits them from their eye specialists. On occasion, illness or emergency treatment may necessitate removal of a person's lenses by the nurse. A hard contact lens wearer who is unconscious and unable to blink can develop corneal abrasions from lack of tears for lubrication. Clients with impaired judgment, eg, from substance abuse, are prone to eye damage from prolonged lens wearing. Careful handling of the lenses by the nurse is essential.

EQUIPMENT

- A lens storage case. Most users have a special container for their lenses. Some contain a solution so that the lenses are stored wet; in others, the lenses are dry. Each lens has a slot with a label indicating whether it is the right or left lens. It is essential that the correct lens be stored in the appropriate slot, since each is ground for a specific eye. The case is placed on the bedside table within easy reach.
    or
  If a lens storage case is not available, two small medicine cups or specimen containers partially filled with normal saline solution. Mark one cup "L lens," the other "R lens."

- A flashlight (optional) to help locate the lens.

- A cotton applicator dipped in saline (optional) to reposition a lens.

- Gloves to protect the nurse.

INTERVENTION

1. Obtain the following information if health permits:
    a. The kind of lenses worn.
    b. When the lenses were prescribed.
    c. When the client last visited an ophthalmologist.
    d. Any problems with either or both eyes or eyelids, such as excessive tearing, burning, redness, sensitivity to light, swelling, or feelings of dryness. (Ask the client to describe them.)
    e. The use of any eyedrops or ointments. (These medications can combine chemically with soft lenses and cause lens damage and eye irritation.)
    f. How often lenses are worn, eg, daily or on special occasions.
    g. The lens-wearing time in a given day, including sleep time.
    h. Whether lenses are alternately worn with eyeglasses.
    i. Whether lenses are removed for certain activities, eg, contact sports or swimming.
    j. Any problems with the lenses, eg, cleaning, insertion, removal, damage.
    k. Whether the client carries an emergency identification label to alert others to remove the lenses and ensure appropriate care. (If not, advise the person to acquire one.)
    l. The insertion and removal procedures.
    m. The cleaning and storage procedures.

2. Inspect the eyes carefully. Pay particular attention to any redness of the conjunctiva or encrustations of the eyelashes.

3. Assist the client to a supine position or a sitting position with the head tilted back.
    Rationale   This prevents the lens from falling onto the floor and causing damage or loss.

4. Don gloves.

5. Locate the position of the lens:
    a. Retract the upper eyelid with your index finger and ask the client to look up, down, and from side to side.
    b. Retract the lower eyelid with your index finger and ask the client to look up and down and from side to side.
    c. Use a flashlight if necessary to find the lens.
    Rationale   Some colorless soft lenses are difficult to see. The lens must be positioned directly over the cornea for proper removal.

6. If the lens is displaced:
    a. Ask the client to look straight ahead.

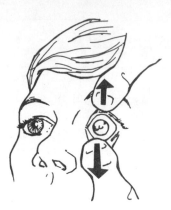

Figure 34–8

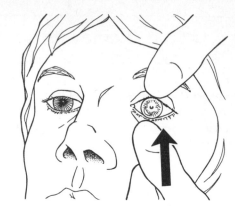

Figure 34–9

b. Using your gloved index fingers, gently exert pressure on the inner margins of the upper and lower lids, and move the lens back onto the cornea.

   or

c. Using a cotton-tipped applicator dipped in saline, gently move the lens into place.

To Remove a Hard Lens

7. After donning gloves, use both thumbs or index fingers to separate the upper and lower eyelids of one eye until they are beyond the edges of the lens. See Figure 34–8. Exert pressure toward the bony orbit above and below the eye.

   Rationale A two-handed method may be needed for clients unable to cooperate. Retraction of the eyelids against the bony orbit prevents direct pressure, discomfort, and injury to the eyeball.

   or

   Use the middle finger to retract the upper eyelid and the thumb of the same hand to retract the lower lid.

   Rationale Using one hand for retraction keeps the other hand free to receive the lens.

8. Gently move the margins of both the lower eyelid and the upper eyelid toward the lens.

   Rationale The margins of the lids trap the edges of the lens.

9. Hold the top eyelid stationary, and lift the bottom edge of the contact lens by pressing the lower lid at its margin firmly under the lens. See Figure 34–9.

   Rationale Pressure exerted under the edge of the lens interrupts the suction of the lens on the cornea. The lens then tips forward at the top edge.

10. Slide the lens off and out of the eye by moving both eyelids toward each other.

11. Grasp the lens with your index finger and thumb and place it in the palm of your hand.

12. Clean according to manufacturer's instructions.

13. Place the lens in the correct slot in its storage case. The slots are labeled for right and left lenses.

14. Repeat steps 7–13 for the other lens.

15. Be sure each lens is centered in the storage case. Tighten or close the cover. Proceed to step 26.

    Rationale If the lens is not centered, it may crack, chip, or tear.

To Remove a Soft Lens

16. Ask the client to look upward at the ceiling and keep the eye opened wide.

17. Retract the lower or upper lid with one or two gloved fingers of your nondominant hand.

18. Using the gloved index finger of your dominant hand, move the lens down to the inferior part of the sclera. See Figure 34–10.

    Rationale Moving the lens onto the sclera reduces the risk of damage to the cornea.

19. Gently pinch the lens between the pads of the thumb and index finger of your dominant hand, and remove the lens. See Figure 34–11.

    Rationale Pinching causes the lens to double up, so that air enters underneath the lens, breaking the suction and allowing removal. The pads of the fingers are used to prevent scratching the eye or the lens with the fingernails.

20. Place the lens in the palm of your hand.

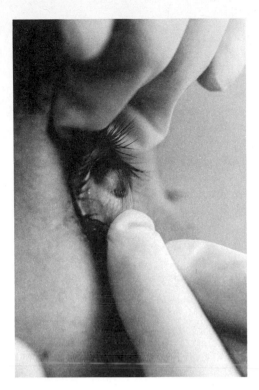

Figure 34–10

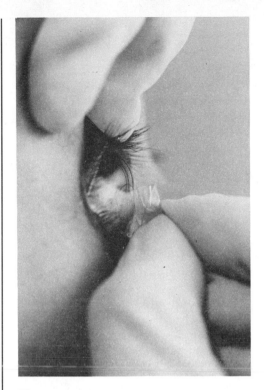

Figure 34–11

21. For ultrathin lenses, open the lens with the thumb and index finger *immediately* upon removal.

    Rationale   It is important to keep the edges from sticking together.

22. Clean according to manufacturer's instructions.

23. Place the lens in the correct slot in its storage case. The slots are labeled for right and left lenses.

24. Repeat steps 16–23 for the other lens.

25. Be sure each lens is centered in the storage case. Tighten or close the cover.

    Rationale   If the lens is not centered, it may crack or tear.

26. Place the contact lens container in the drawer of the bedside table.

Rationale   The lenses and the case should never be exposed to direct sunlight or extreme heat, since these can dry or warp them.

27. Document the removal of the lenses prior to surgery or when this is a nursing responsibility. Document all assessments and problems, such as redness of the conjunctiva, and report problems to the nurse in charge.

Sample Recording

Date	Time	Notes
3/22/89	2100	Contact lenses removed. No redness of the conjunctiva noted. ———————— ————————Anita R. Rodriguez, SN

PROCEDURE 34–12 **Cleaning Contact Lenses (Hard and Soft)**

Contact lenses need to be cleaned in a sterile, non-irritating wetting solution before they are inserted. The wetting solution helps the lens to glide over the cornea, thus reducing the risk of injury. Some people use their saliva to wet their lenses. Such practices need to be discouraged, since contaminants in saliva can cause bacterial buildup on the lens. Such a buildup can lead to infection.

Lenses are cleaned relatively easily with chemical lens-cleaning solutions provided with the lenses. Soft lenses can also be cleaned by electric heat disinfecting units. In addition to regular heat disinfection, soft lenses need to be cleaned weekly with an enzymatic solution that dissolves protein deposits. Proper storage of lenses is essential. Soft lenses can become dry, brittle, and permanently damaged if left exposed to the air for an hour or less. Sterile saline is the preferred storage solution, since unsterile solutions facilitate bacterial growth, and the minerals present in tap water can damage a soft lens.

EQUIPMENT

- The client's lens storage case and lenses.
- Gloves to protect the nurse.

For Hard Lenses

- Contact lens cleaner. This is usually a sterile, antiseptic nonirritating solution labeled "lens cleaner."
- An absorbent applicator or cotton balls for spreading the cleaning solution (optional).
- Warm water.
- Soaking solution (optional).

For Soft Lenses: Heat Disinfection

- A heat disinfecting case.
- Saline solution (a salt tablet and distilled water).
- Cleaning solution (prepared from an enzyme tablet and distilled water).

For Soft Lenses: Chemical Disinfection

- Lens-cleaning solution.

- Rinsing solution.
- Disinfection and storage solution.

INTERVENTION

1. Don gloves.

2. Open the lens container carefully.

   Rationale Soft contact lenses tend to pop out unexpectedly when the case is opened quickly.

3. Pick up one lens from the container.

   Rationale The lenses are cleaned one at a time to make sure they are not put in the wrong slot or wrong eye.

4. Inspect the lenses for scratches or tears and determine the client's cleaning and storage practices.

To Clean Hard Lenses

5. Wet the lens by placing a few drops of lens cleaner on both sides of it.

6. Spread the solution on both surfaces with the thumb and index finger or an absorbent applicator, or place the lens in the palm of your hand and spread the solution with your index finger.

   Rationale The solution removes dirt and film.

7. Position the lens on the palm side of the index or middle finger.

8. Rinse the lens with warm tap water that feels comfortable to the fingers. If the tap water contains excessive chlorine or minerals, use distilled or purified water. If rinsing the lens over a sink, be sure the sink drain is closed.

   Rationale Hot water is contraindicated because plastic will warp when exposed to extreme heat. The closer the lens is to body temperature the more comfortable it will feel on insertion. While rinsing removes dirt, it is not necessary to rinse away all of the lens cleaner since this agent has beneficial sterilizing and wetting properties. A closed sink drain prevents the lenses from being lost down the drain.

9. Place the lens in a soaking solution or store it dry, in accordance with the recommendations of the client's physician.

10. Follow steps 5–9 to clean the second lens.

To Clean Soft Lenses by Chemical Disinfection

11. Place a few drops of lens cleaner on both sides of the lens and spread it as described in step 6.

12. Position the lens as described in step 7.

13. Rinse the lens thoroughly with rinsing solution.

14. Place the lens in the correct slot of the storage area.

15. Fill the slot with storage and disinfectant solution and tightly close its cap.

16. Follow steps 11–15 for the other lens.

17. Store both lenses for at least 4 hours.

18. Clean and rinse the lenses before insertion. Follow steps 11–13.

19. Clean the storage slots by emptying the solution and rinsing them with hot water and rinsing solution. Allow them to air dry.

To Clean Soft Lenses by Heat Disinfection

20. Put a few drops of normal saline solution on each lens and spread it on the lens as described in step 6.

21. Rinse the lenses thoroughly with tap water.

22. Place each lens in the appropriate slot of the heat disinfecting unit, and fill the slots with normal saline solution.

23. Make sure the disinfecting unit is placed on a heat-resistant surface. Plug the unit into an electric outlet, and turn it on. The unit will turn off automatically after disinfection is completed.

To Clean Soft Lenses with an Enzymatic Solution (Weekly)

24. Rinse and fill the plastic or glass wells of the lens storage case with distilled water.

25. Place an enzymatic cleaning tablet in each well.

26. Place one lens in each well and securely close the caps.

27. Shake the wells to dissolve the tablets.

28. Soak the lenses for 6–12 hours or overnight.

29. Remove the lenses, and thoroughly rinse them with saline solution.

30. Place the lenses in the heat disinfecting unit and follow steps 22–23.

31. Rinse the storage wells with tap water, and allow them to air dry.

32. Document cleaning of the lenses with removal or insertion of the lenses.

PROCEDURE 34-13 **Inserting Contact Lenses (Hard and Soft)**

Seriously ill people who have had their contact lenses removed will not need them reinserted until they become more active in their care and require their lenses to see. When assisting the client with lens reinsertion, the nurse must ensure that the lenses are adequately cleaned. See Procedure 34-12.

EQUIPMENT

- The client's lens storage case.

- A wetting agent to lubricate the lenses. Solutions of methyl cellulose or polyvinyl alcohol are frequently used.

- Gloves to protect the nurse.

INTERVENTION

1. Don gloves and inspect the lenses for cleanliness, scratches, and tears.

2. Inspect the eyes for redness of the conjunctiva, encrustations of the eyelashes, or any other problems.

3. Ensure that the correct lens is selected for the eye. It is always wise to start with the right eye.

   Rationale Each lens is ground to fit the individual eye and correct its visual defect. Always starting with the right eye establishes a habit so that incorrect placement of each lens is avoided.

To Insert Hard Lenses

4. Put a few drops of wetting solution on the right lens.

   Rationale Wetting solution lubricates the lens, facilitates insertion, and lessens the chance of damage to the eye.

5. Spread the wetting solution on both surfaces of the lens by using your thumb and index finger, or place the lens in the palm of your hand and spread the solution with your index finger.

6. Place the lens convex side down on the tip of your dominant index finger (the right, if you are righthanded). See Figure 34-12.

7. Ask the client to bend the head backward.

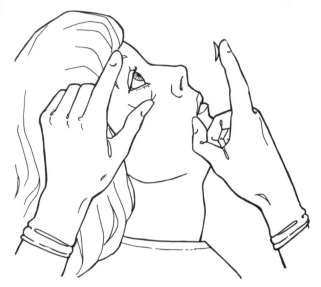

Figure 34-12

8. Separate the upper and lower eyelids of the right eye with the thumb and index finger of your non-dominant hand. See Figure 34-12. Place your thumb on the skin over the infraorbital bone, your index finger on the skin over the supraorbital bone.

   Rationale Retraction of the eyelids against the bony orbit prevents direct pressure, discomfort, and injury to the eyeball.

9. Place the lens as gently as possible on the cornea, directly over the iris and pupil.

10. Ask whether the vision is blurred following insertion.

    Rationale If vision is blurred, the lens may be off center.

11. If so, center the lens as follows.

    a. Separate the eyelids by using the index or middle finger of the left hand to lift the upper lid and the index or middle finger of the right hand to depress the lower lid. See Figure 34-13.

    b. Locate the lens, and ask the client to gaze in the opposite direction. See Figure 34-13.

    c. Gently push the lens in the direction of the cornea, using a finger or the eyelid margins.

    d. Ask the client to look slowly toward the lens. The lens will slide easily onto the cornea.

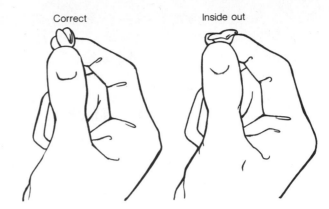

Figure 34-15

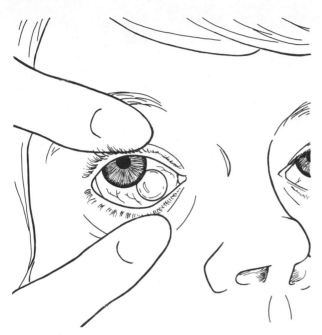

Figure 34-13

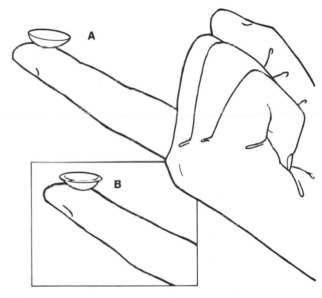

Figure 34-16

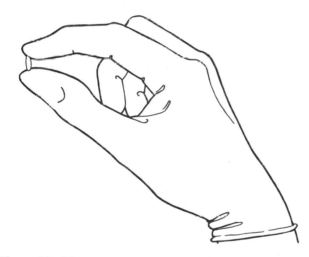

Figure 34-14

12. Repeat steps 4–11 for the other lens. Then proceed to step 23.

To Insert Soft Lenses

13. Remove the lens from its saline-filled storage case with your nondominant hand. If the lens is ultrathin, allow it to air dry for a few seconds.

    Rationale   The dominant fingers must be kept dry for inserting the lens.

14. To position a regular (not ultrathin) lens correctly for insertion:

a. Hold the lens at the edge between your thumb and index finger. See Figure 34–14.

b. Flex the lens slightly. The lens is in the correct position if the edges point inward. It is in the wrong position (ie, inside out) and must be reversed if the edges point outward. See Figure 34–15.

    Rationale   A lens placed on the eye inside out is less comfortable (an edge sensation may be felt), tends to fold on the eye, can drop to a lower position on the eye, and may move excessively on blinking.

15. Do *not* flex an ultrathin lens. Instead, put the lens on your placement finger and allow it to dry slightly for a few seconds. Closely inspect the lens to see if the edges turn upward, as shown in Figure 34–16, A. If they turn downward, as shown

in Figure 34–16, B, the lens is inside out and must be reversed.

Rationale   Flexing an ultrathin lens may cause the lens to fold and stick together.

16. Wet the lens with saline solution as described in step 4, using your nondominant fingers.

17. Ensure that your placement finger is dry. This is particularly important for ultrathin soft lenses.

    Rationale   "Water-loving" soft contact lenses have a natural attraction to wet surfaces. Insertion onto the moist eye is facilitated when the finger is dry.

18. Place the lens convex side down on the tip of your dominant index finger.

    Rationale   The concave side of the lens rests against the cornea.

19. Keep the lens parallel with the fingertip, with all edges up and toward the eye. See Figure 34–16, A.

    Rationale   Balancing the lens in an upright position facilitates insertion. A lens that rocks forward or sideways, allowing one edge to touch the fingertip, hinders insertion.

20. If the lens curls and the edges stick together, place the lens in the palm of your hand, wet it thoroughly with saline solution, and gently move the edges apart by rubbing the lens between your thumb and index finger, or soak the lens in saline solution.

21. If the lens flattens or drapes across the finger, move the lens to the palm of your nondominant hand, dry the placement finger, and allow the lens to air dry for a few seconds.

    Rationale   The placement finger or the lens may be too wet.

22. Follow steps 7–9 above for insertion.

23. Replace the lens container, lens cleaner, and wetting solution in the drawer of the bedside table.

24. Document insertion of the contact lenses if a nurse is required to remove them; otherwise, this is not normally recorded (consult agency policy). Document all assessments and report to the nurse in charge any problems observed in the eyes or the lenses.

25. Document on the nursing care plan the time for the lenses to be removed.

PROCEDURE 34–14 **Removing, Cleaning, and Inserting a Hearing Aid**

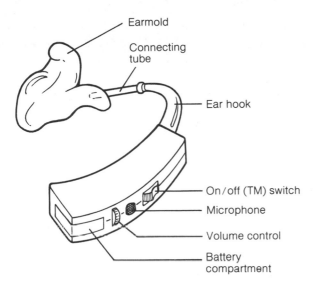

Figure 34–17
A behind-the-ear hearing aid.

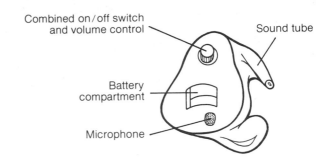

Figure 34–18
An in-the-ear hearing aid.

A hearing aid is a battery-powered sound-amplifying device used by hearing-impaired persons. It consists of a microphone that picks up the sound and converts it to electric energy, an amplifier that magnifies the electric energy electronically, a receiver that converts the amplified energy back to sound energy, and an earmold that directs the sound into the ear. The on/off switch may be designated as "O" (off), "M" microphone, "T" (telephone), or "TM" (telephone/microphone). There are several types of hearing aids:

- *Behind-the-ear-aid:* This is the most widely used type, since it fits snugly over the ear. The hearing aid case, which holds the microphone, amplifier, and receiver is attached to the earmold by a plastic tube. See Figure 34–17.

- *In-the-ear-aid:* This one-piece aid is the most compact hearing aid. All its components are housed in the earmold. Because this is the least powerful aid, it is recommended for only the mildly impaired person. See Figure 34–18.

- *Eyeglasses aid:* This is similar to the behind-the-ear aid except that the components are housed in the temple of the eyeglasses. The hearing aid can be in one or both temples of the glasses. See Figure 34–19. An eyeglasses aid is useful for what is referred to as the contralateral routing of signals (CROS). Sounds entering the impaired ear are amplified and redirected to the good ear.

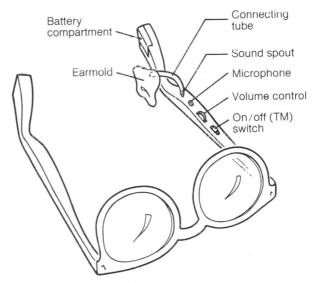

Figure 34–19
An eyeglasses hearing aid.

- *Body hearing aid:* This pocket-sized aid, used for more severe hearing losses, clips onto an undergarment, shirt pocket, or harness carrier supplied by the manufacturer. See Figure 34–20. The case, containing the microphone and large amplifier, is connected by a cord to the receiver, which snaps into the earpiece.

For correct functioning, hearing aids require appropriate handling during insertion and removal, regular cleaning of the earmold, and replacement of dead batteries. With proper care hearing aids generally last 5–10 years. Earmolds generally need readjustment every 2–3 years.

Although most people can look after their hearing aids themselves, some debilitated individuals may

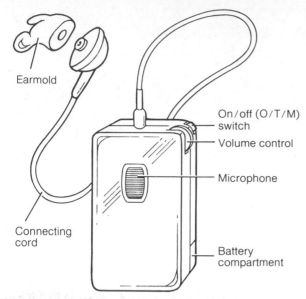

Earmold

On/off (O/T/M) switch

Volume control

Microphone

Connecting cord

Battery compartment

Figure 34-20
A body hearing aid.

require assistance. Hearing aids must be removed before surgery.

EQUIPMENT

- The hearing aid.
- A new battery (if needed).
- A pipe cleaner or toothpick (optional).
- Soap, water, and towels or a damp cloth.
- Gloves to protect the nurse.

INTERVENTION

1. Determine
   a. The type of hearing aid worn
   b. When and where it was obtained and from whom
   c. Maintenance and cleaning methods
   d. Any hearing aid problems
   e. Any ear problems

Removing a Hearing Aid

2. Turn the hearing aid off and lower the volume.
   Rationale The batteries continue to be used if the aid is not turned off.

3. Don gloves and remove the earmold by rotating it slightly forward and pulling it outward.

4. If the aid is not to be used for several days, remove the battery.
   Rationale Removal prevents corrosion of the aid from battery leakage.

5. Store the hearing aid in a safe place. Avoid exposure to heat, moisture, sprays, and aerosols.
   Rationale Safe storage prevents loss or damage.

Cleaning the Earmold

6. Detach the earmold *if possible.* Disconnect the earmold from the receiver of a body hearing aid or from the hearing aid case of behind-the-ear and eyeglasses aids where the tubing meets the hook of the case. Do not remove the earmold if it is glued or secured by a small metal ring.
   Rationale Removal facilitates cleaning the earmold and prevents inadvertent damage to the other parts.

7. If the earmold is detachable, soak it in a mild soapy solution. Rinse and dry it well. Never use alcohol for cleaning. It can dry and crack the mold.

8. If the earmold is not detachable or for an in-the-ear aid, wipe the ear mold with a damp cloth.

9. Ensure that the earmold opening is patent. Blow any excess moisture through the opening or remove debris (eg, earwax) with a pipe cleaner or toothpick.

10. Reattach the earmold if it was detached from the rest of the hearing aid.

Inserting the Hearing Aid

11. Determine from the client whether the earmold is for the left or the right ear.

12. Check that the battery is inserted in the hearing aid.

13. Turn off the hearing aid, and make sure the volume is turned all the way down.

14. Inspect the earmold to identify the ear canal portion.
    Rationale Some earmolds are fitted for only the ear canal and *concha*; others are fitted for all the contours of the ear. The canal portion, common to all, can be used as a guide for correct insertion.

15. Line up the parts of the earmold with the corresponding parts of the client's ear.

16. Rotate the earmold slightly forward and insert the ear canal portion.

17. Gently press the earmold into the ear while rotating it backward.

18. Check that the earmold fits snugly by asking the client if it feels secure and comfortable.

19. Adjust the other components of a behind-the-ear or body hearing aid.

20. Turn the hearing aid on and adjust the volume according to the person's needs.

21. If the hearing aid is not functioning properly, ie, the sound is weak or there is no sound:

    a. Ensure that the volume is turned high enough.

    b. Ensure that the earmold opening is not clogged.

    c. Check the battery, by turning the aid on, turning up the volume, cupping your hand over the earmold, and listening. A constant whistling sound indicates the battery is functioning. If necessary, replace the battery. Be sure to match the negative (−) and positive (+) signs when inserting the new battery.

    d. Ensure that the ear canal is not blocked with wax, which can obstruct sound waves.

22. If the person reports a whistling sound or squeal after insertion:

    a. Turn the volume down.

    b. Ensure that the earmold is properly attached to the receiver.

    c. Reinsert the earmold.

23. When communicating, be sure to face the client, and talk distinctly in natural tones. Do not shout.

    Rationale   Facing the person directly facilitates lip reading by some people. Natural tones are more easily amplified.

24. Document and record nursing assessments and interventions. Removal and insertion of a hearing aid are not normally recorded.

Considerations for the Elderly

Elderly people need time to adjust to hearing aids, since they amplify all sounds even background noise. Therefore, when talking with persons with hearing aids the nurse needs to keep away from distractions such as a television or other conversations, select a quiet area, and talk in slow normal tones. First-time wearers need to use their hearing aids for only 1 hour a day initially and gradually increase the time to 12 hours a day.

PROCEDURE 34–15   **Changing an Occupied Bed**

Not all clients are able to leave their beds. Those who cannot must remain in bed when the linen is changed. In most acute care hospitals, the beds are made once a day. The linen is changed at that time and whenever it becomes soiled. Long-term and nonacute agencies change bed linens less often. Use the following guidelines when making an occupied bed:

- Maintain the client in good body alignment.

- Move the client gently, smoothly, and appropriately for the condition. Rough handling can cause the client discomfort and abrade the skin.

- Throughout the procedure, explain what you plan to do before you do it. Use terms that the person can understand.

- Never move or position a client in a manner that is contraindicated for health, comfort, or safety. For example, the client who is dyspneic should be maintained in Fowler's position and not placed in a supine position.

- Use the bedmaking time, like the bed bath time, to assess and meet the client's needs (eg, the need for information about a forthcoming operation).

Hospital beds are often changed after bed baths. The linen can be collected before the bath. Some hospitals do not change linen unless it is soiled.

EQUIPMENT

The following equipment is usually required for a complete bed change:

- A mattress pad, if necessary
- Two large sheets
- A bedspread
- A waterproof pad, if required
- A cloth drawsheet
- Two pillowcases
- Bath blanket (optional)

INTERVENTION

1. Determine the movement and the positions the client can assume in accordance with health status.

2. Make significant health assessments appropriate for the client, eg, pulse, respirations, color.

3. Place the fresh linen on the bedside chair or overbed table within easy reach and in order of use.

4. Remove any equipment attached to the bed linen, such as a signal light.

Removing the Top Bedding

5. Loosen all the top linen at the foot of the bed.

6. Using both hands, grasp the top edge of the spread, one hand at the center, the other at the mattress edge. Fold it in half by bringing the top edge even with the bottom edge.
   Rationale   Linens folded this way are readily reapplied to the bed later.

7. Pick up the spread carefully by grasping it at the center of the middle fold and the bottom edges.

8. If the spread is soiled, place it in the linen hamper or tuck it in at the bottom of the bed. Some agencies have portable linen hampers that can be taken to the bed unit. If the agency has a central disposal chute for linen, collect all the soiled linen at the foot of the bed to take to the chute. Take care to prevent the soiled linen from touching your uniform.
   Rationale   The uniform can become soiled and transmit microorganisms to others.

9. If the spread is not soiled and is to be reused, lay it over the back of the bedside chair.

10. Repeat steps 6–9 for the blanket.

11. Leave the top sheet over the client (the top sheet can remain in place if it is being discarded and if it will provide sufficient warmth)
    or
    replace it with a bath blanket as follows:
    a. Spread the bath blanket over the top sheet.
    b. Ask the client to hold the top edge of the blanket.
    c. Reaching under the blanket from the side, grasp the top edge of the sheet and draw it down to the foot of the bed, leaving the blanket in place.
    d. Remove the sheet from the bed and place it with the soiled linen.

Moving the Mattress Up on the Bed

12. Place the bed in the flat position if the client's health permits.

13. Loosen the foundation on the near side to expose the mattress.

14. Grasp the mattress lugs and, using good body mechanics, move the mattress up to the head of the bed. Ask the client to assist, if permitted, by grasping the head of the bed and pulling as you push. If the client is heavy, you may need help from another nurse.

    Rationale   When the head of the bed is raised, the mattress tends to slide toward the foot of the bed, thus moving the client toward the foot of the bed.

Changing the Foundation of the Bed

15. Assist the client to turn on a side, facing away from the linen supply and on the far side of the bed. Raise the side rail on the far side.

    Rationale   This leaves the near half of the foundation free to be changed. The raised side rail protects the client from falling. If there is no side rail, have another nurse support the client at the edge of the bed.

16. Returning to the first side of the bed, loosen the foundation linen at the side. Remove or fanfold the waterproof pad if used. Fanfold the drawsheet and the bottom sheet at the center of the bed, as close to the client as possible.

    Rationale   Close fanfolding makes room for the new linen.

17. Smooth the mattress pad, if it is to be retained. If not, fanfold it, and place a new pad on the bed, with the center fold at the center of the bed and the uppermost half fanfolded at the center.

    Rationale   Smoothing removes wrinkles that could irritate the client's skin.

18. Place the new bottom sheet on the bed so that the lower edge extends slightly, eg, 2.5 cm (1 in.), over the end of the mattress. Make sure that the hem of the sheet is facing down.

    Rationale   The hem edge can irritate the client's skin.

19. Moving from the foot to the head, open the sheet lengthwise.

20. Fanfold the uppermost half of the clean bottom sheet vertically at the center of the bed.

21. Tuck the sheet under the near half of the head of the bed. Miter the sheet at the top corner of the side of the bed or fit the corner of a contour sheet under the mattress.

    Rationale   A mitered corner holds the sheet firmly in place.

22. Moving toward the foot of the bed, tuck the bottom sheet under the side of the mattress, smoothing the sheet at the same time.

    Rationale   Wrinkles could irritate the client's skin.

23. Pull the cloth drawsheet from the center of the bed, where it was fanfolded. Tuck it under the side of the mattress. If a clean drawsheet is to be used:

    a. Lay it on the bed with the center fold at the center of the bed. The drawsheet should extend from midway down the client's back to midway down the thighs.

    b. Fanfold the uppermost half vertically at the center of the bed.

    c. Tuck the near side edge under the side of the mattress.

24. Make sure waterproof pad, if used, is under the client's buttocks.

25. Assist the client to roll over toward you onto the clean side of the bed. The client rolls over the fanfolded linen at the center of the bed.

26. Move the pillows to the clean side for the client. The cases should be changed at this point if they are soiled.

    Rationale   Pillows provide support.

27. Raise the side rail, if necessary, before leaving the side of the bed.

    Rationale   The side rail provides safety and a sense of security for the client.

28. Move to the other side of the bed and lower the side rail if one is being used.

29. Loosen the foundation linen on that side. Fanfold the drawsheets if they are being reused, and remove the soiled bottom sheet. Remove the drawsheets with the bottom sheet if they are being changed. Roll the linens so that the client does not see the soiled parts.

    Rationale   Sight of the soil might be embarrassing to the person.

30. Place the soiled linen at the foot of the bed or in the portable linen hamper.

Rationale   This helps to prevent the spread of microorganisms contained in linens soiled with the client's excretions or other body discharges.

31. Smooth out the mattress cover to remove any wrinkles.

32. Unfold the fanfolded bottom sheet from the center of the bed.

33. Tuck the top of the sheet under the near half of the head of the bed. Miter the sheet at the top corner of the side of the bed.

34. Facing the side of the bed, use both hands to pull the bottom sheet so that it is smooth, and tuck the excess under the side of the mattress. See Figure 34–21.

    Rationale   Pulling at an angle removes wrinkles.

35. Unfold the cloth drawsheet fanfolded at the center of the bed, and pull it tightly with both hands. Pull the sheet in three sections: Face the side of the bed to pull the middle section, face the far top corner to pull the bottom section, and face the far bottom corner to pull the top section. Tuck the excess sheet under the side of the mattress.

36. Smooth out the waterproof pad.

37. Reposition the pillows at the center of the bed.

38. Assist the client to the center of the bed and to the position preferred or required.

39. Raise the side rail on the second side of the bed, if required, and return to the first side. Lower the side rail on the first side.

Making the Top of the Bed

40. Spread the top sheet over the client so that the center crease is in the center of the bed and the top edge is at the client's shoulders. There should be enough sheet at the top so that a cuff can be folded over the blanket and spread.

41. Ask the client to hold the top edge of the sheet or tuck it under the shoulders. The sheet should remain over the client when the bath blanket or used sheet is removed.

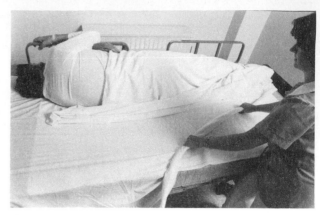

Figure 34–21

42. Reaching under the fresh sheet, grasp the bottom edge of the bath blanket or used sheet and remove it by pulling it to the foot of the bed.

43. Fold the bath blanket and put it in the bedside table if it is to be reused, or place the used sheet with the soiled linen.

44. Complete the top of the bed as for an unoccupied bed.

45. Attach the signal cord to the bed linen within the client's reach. Some cords have clamps that attach to the sheet or pillowcase; others are attached by a safety pin.

46. Put the bedside table and the overbed table in order. Put items used by the client within easy reach.

47. Adjust the side rails and the height of the bed for the client's needs and according to agency policy. Some hospitals require that the side rails be raised for all people 70 years old and older and that all beds be left in the low position.

48. Document pertinent assessment data. Changing bed linen is not normally recorded.

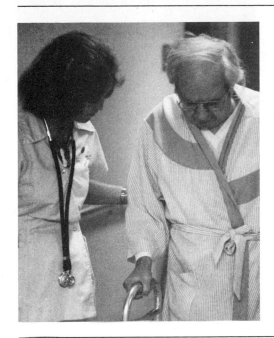

CHAPTER 35

MOBILITY AND IMMOBILITY

☐ The following procedures appear in
Introduction to Nursing:

Procedure 35–1
Providing Passive Range-of-Motion Exercises

■ New procedure:

Procedure 35–2
Applying Restraints

PROCEDURE 35–2   **Applying Restraints**

EQUIPMENT

Select the kind and size of restraint required by the client. Before selecting a restraint, nurses need to understand its purpose clearly. Then they can choose a restraint that best meets the needs of the client. Restraints should be measured against the following criteria in the process of selection:

- Does it restrict the client's movement as little as possible?

- Does it restrain more than is necessary? For example, if a person needs to have one arm restrained, do not restrain the entire body.

- Is it the least obvious to others? Both clients and support persons are often embarrassed by a restraint, even though they understand why it is being used. The less obvious the restraint, the more comfortable people feel. For example, a crossover jacket restraint may be less conspicuous than arm and leg restraints.

- Does it interfere with the client's therapy or health? For example, if a person has impaired blood circulation to the hands, apply a restraint that will not aggravate that circulatory problem.

- Is it readily changeable? Restraints need to be changed frequently (see the next section), and more often if they become soiled. Keeping other guidelines in mind, choose a restraint that can be changed with minimal disturbance to the client.

- Is it safe for the particular client? Choose a restraint with which the client cannot self-inflict injury. For example, a physically active child could incur injury trying to climb out of a crib if one wrist is tied to the side of the crib. A jacket restraint would restrain the child more safely.

If a commercial hand, wrist, or ankle restraint is not available, the supplies that follow are needed.

Mitt restraint:

- Four large padded dressings, eg, ABD pads

- Pieces of thick gauze to put between the person's fingers

- A stockinette dressing or elastic bandage

- Adhesive tape

Wrist or ankle restraint:

- A padded or thick gauze dressing, eg, an ABD pad

- A strip of gauze bandage or cloth tie 5–8 cm (2–3 in.) wide and 90–120 cm (3–4 ft) long

INTERVENTION

1. Assess client's level of consciousness and condition of skin in area to be restrained.

2. Explain to the client and support persons how the restraint is used and its purpose. Give the explanation even to disoriented and unconscious people; they may understand what you are saying.

Jacket Restraint

3. Put the jacket on over the client's gown and bring the ties to the sides.

4. Ensure that the gown and the jacket are not wrinkled.
   Rationale Wrinkles could irritate the skin.

5. Using a half-bow knot, secure each tie to the part of the bed frame that moves when the head is elevated. See Figure 35–1.
   Rationale If tied to the movable part of the bed frame, the jacket will not tighten when the bed is elevated. The half-bow knot does not tighten or slip when the attached end is pulled but unties easily when the loose end is pulled.

Belt Restraint (Safety Belt)

6. Determine that the safety belt is in good order. If a Velcro safety belt is to be used, make sure that both pieces of Velcro are intact.

7. Place the long portion of the belt behind (under) the client and secure it to the movable part of the bed frame.
   Rationale The long attached portion will then move up when the head of the bed is elevated and will not tighten around the client.

8. Place the shorter portion of the belt around the client's waist, over the gown. There should be a finger's width between the belt and the client.

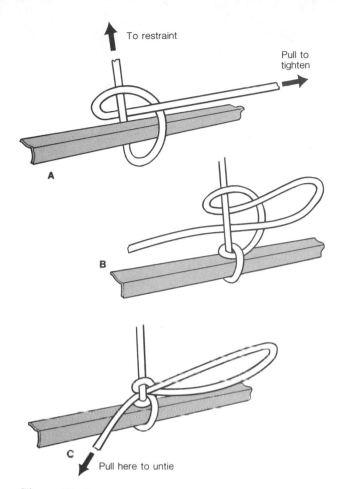

Figure 35-1
Tying a half-bow knot.

Mitt Restraint

9. Apply the mitt to the hand to be restrained. Make sure the fingers can be slightly flexed and are not caught under the hand. Some clients may require only one restraint, eg, if the other hand is paralyzed or already secured by a wrist restraint for an IV.

10. If there is no commercial mitt, make a mitt as follows:

   a. Place a large folded dressing, such as an abdominal (ABD) pad, in the client's palm. Ensure that the hand is in a natural position with the fingers slightly flexed.

   b. Separate the fingers with pieces of large dressing or thick gauze, to prevent skin abrasion.

   c. Put a padded dressing around the client's wrist to prevent pressure and skin abrasion.

   d. Place two large dressings (ABD pads) over the hand. Place the first one from the back of the

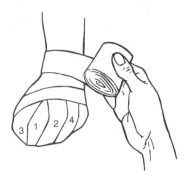

Figure 35-2

hand over the fingers to the palm; then wrap the other from side to side around the hand.

   e. Cover these dressings by placing a stockinette dressing over the hand or wrapping them with an elastic bandage, using a recurrent pattern. See Figure 35-2.

   f. Secure the stockinette or elastic bandage with adhesive tape.

11. If a mitt is to be worn for several days, remove it at least every 12 hours. Wash and exercise the client's hand, then reapply the mitt. Check agency practices about recommended intervals for removal. Assess the client's circulation to the hands shortly after the mitt is applied and at regular intervals. Feelings of numbness, discomfort, or inability to move the fingers could indicate impaired circulation to the hand.

Wrist or Ankle Restraint

12. Apply the padded portion of a commercially prepared restraint around the ankle or wrist
   or
   Improvise a restraint as follows:

   a. Cushion the wrist or ankle with a padded or thick gauze dressing, eg, an ABD pad.

   b. Wrap a long, narrow strip of gauze bandage or a cloth tie around the padding.

13. Pull the tie of the commercially made restraint through the slit in the wrist portion or through the buckle
   or
   Use a clove hitch to secure the gauze strip or cloth tie of the improvised restraint. See Figure 35-3.

14. Using a half-bow knot or a square knot as appropriate, attach the other end of the commercial restraint (or the two ends of the improvised

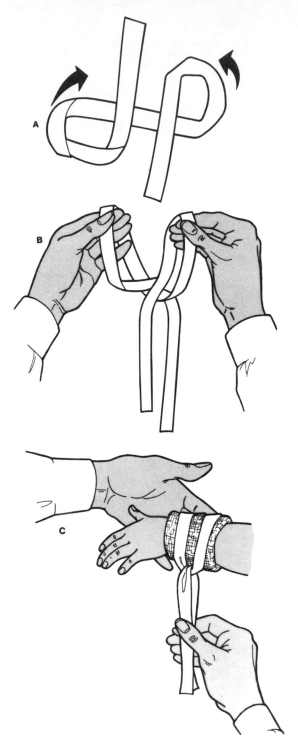

Figure 35–3
Making a clove-hitch restraint.

restraint) to the movable portion of the bed frame. See figures 35–1 and 35–4 for how to tie these knots.

Rationale If the ties are attached to the movable portion of the bed frame, the wrist or ankle will not be pulled when the bed position is changed.

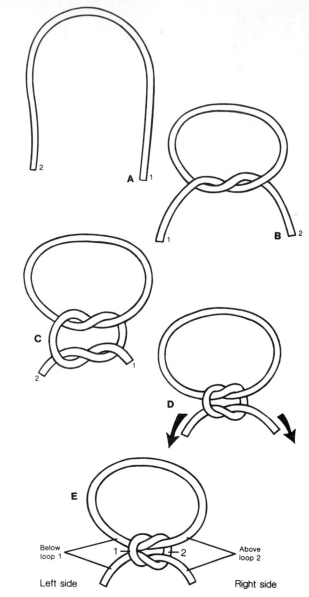

Figure 35–4
Tying a square (reef) knot.

15. Ensure that restraint placement does not interfere with side rail functioning. Never tie a restraint to a side rail.

    Rationale Lowering the side rail with an attached restraint would tighten the restraint.

16. Adjust the nursing care plan as required, eg, to include releasing the restraint, providing skin care, and providing ROM exercises.

17. Document all assessments and interventions. Also document the need to discuss the restraint with the support persons if it has not already been discussed.

Sample Recording

Date	Time	Notes
9/29/89	0320	Found climbing over side rails. Explained possibility of falling and injury. Sat with client for 10 minutes. She continued to try to climb over side rails. Stated "Don't know where I am."
	0330	Jacket restraint applied. Dr. Singh notified. —————Edward R. King, NS
	0345	Daughter with client. Resting more comfortably. Restraint removed.———
	0400	130 ml clear fluid taken. Voided.——— —————————Edward R. King, NS

Considerations for the Elderly

When hospitalization occurs along with its unfamiliar surroundings, an elderly person may be confused. Nurses can often offer reassurance, calm the client, and restore psychologic comfort by listening to concerns and spending a few minutes at the bedside. In many instances the need for restraining devices can be eliminated. The nurse plays an important role in discovering possible sources of what may be perceived to be unsafe behavior and, in so doing, reducing the need for restraints.

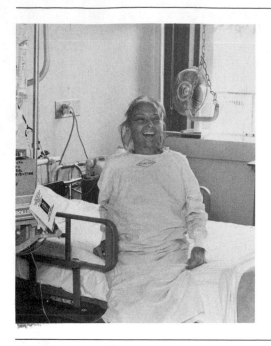

BODY MECHANICS, AMBULATION, AND ALIGNMENT

PROCEDURE 36–7 **Making and Applying a Trochanter Roll**

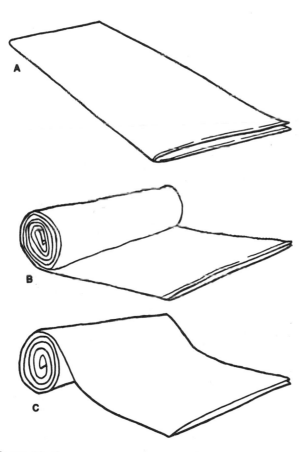

Figure 36–1

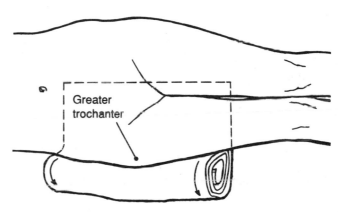

Figure 36–2

A trochanter roll is a roll of cloth, frequently a towel, that is placed against the greater trochanter of the femur to prevent external rotation of the hip. Trochanter rolls are made commercially or can be constructed as described here. A commercial roll needs only to be covered before it is used.

EQUIPMENT

- A bath towel or towel-sized cloth

INTERVENTION

1. Fold the bath towel in half lengthwise. See Figure 36–1, A.

2. Roll the towel tightly, starting at one narrow edge and rolling to within about 30 cm (1 ft) of the other edge. See Figure 36–1, B.

3. Invert the roll. See Figure 36–1, C.

4. Place the flat part of the towel under the client's hip. See Figure 36–2.

5. Turn the roll under and position it tightly against the greater trochanter until the client's toes point directly upward, ie, until the hip is neither externally nor internally rotated.

6. Repeat for the other leg if required.

PROCEDURE 36–8 **Supporting a Client in Lateral Position**

In the lateral (side-lying) position, the body weight is borne by the greater tubercle of the humerus, the acromial process of the clavicle, the ischium, and the greater trochanter of the femur. Both arms lie in front of the client. See Figure 36–3. If appropriate supportive devices are used, this is a comfortable position and a welcome change for the person who has been lying in the prone or supine position for a period of time. The major disadvantage is the tendency for the shoulders and uppermost thigh to rotate inward.

EQUIPMENT

- Up to five small pillows
- A folded towel (optional)

INTERVENTION

1. Assist the client to a lateral position.

2. Place a pillow under the client's head to align the head and neck with the trunk.

   Rationale This pillow prevents lateral flexion and discomfort of the major neck muscles, the sternocleidomastoid muscles.

3. Have the client flex the lower shoulder, position it forward so that the body does not rest on it, and rotate it into any position of comfort so that circulation is not disrupted.

4. Place a pillow under the upper arm.

   Rationale This pillow prevents internal rotation and adduction of the shoulder and downward pressure on the chest that could interfere with chest expansion during respiration. If the client has respiratory difficulty, increase the shoulder flexion and position the upper arm in front of the body off the chest.

5. Place two or more pillows under the upper leg and thigh so that the extremity lies in a plane parallel to the surface of the bed.

   Rationale A position parallel to the bed most closely approximates correct standing alignment and prevents internal rotation of the thigh and adduction of the leg. The pillow also prevents pressure caused by the weight of the top leg resting on the lower leg. Such pressure can damage the vein walls in the lower leg and predispose the client to thrombus formation.

6. Ensure that the two shoulders are aligned in the same plane as the two hips. If they are not, pull one shoulder or hip forward or backward until all four joints are aligned in the same plane.

   Rationale Proper alignment prevents twisting of the spine.

7. Place a folded towel under the natural hollow at the waistline. Take care to fill in only the space at the waistline (optional).

   Rationale A folded towel prevents postural scoliosis of the lumbar spine. A towel support that extends too high or too low creates undue pressure against the rib cage or iliac crests.

8. Place a rolled pillow at the client's back to stabilize the position (optional). This pillow is not usually needed when the client's upper hip and knee are appropriately flexed.

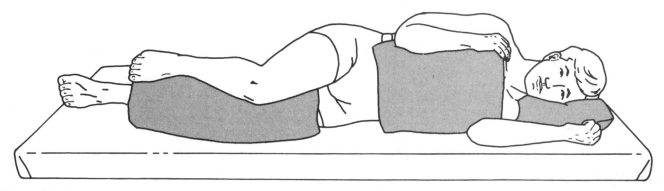

Figure 36–3
Lateral position (supported).

| PROCEDURE 36–9 | **Moving a Client Up in Bed** |

Moving a client up toward the head of the bed is facilitated if the person can safely tolerate having the head of the bed lowered to a flat position and the head pillow removed for a few minutes. If this is not possible, it is wise to obtain a second person to help from the other side of the bed. With this assistance the client will experience less exertion and less discomfort. The steps presented here are followed by either one or two nurses.

INTERVENTION

1. Obtain assessment data.

2. Adjust the head of the bed to a flat position or make it as low as the client can tolerate.

   Rationale The client then does not have to move against gravity.

3. Raise the bed to the height of the nurse's center of gravity and lock the wheels on the bed. Raise the rail on the side of the bed opposite the nurse.

4. Remove all pillows; then place one at the head of the bed.

   Rationale The pillow will protect the client's head from inadvertent injury against the top of the bed.

5. Ask the client to flex the hips and knees and position the feet so that they can be used effectively for pushing.

   Rationale Flexing the hips and knees keeps the entire lower leg off the bed surface, preventing friction during movement. Flexing the hips and knees ensures use of the large muscle groups in the client's legs when pushing and increases the force of movement. The client is encouraged to assist as much as possible with movement to lessen the workload of the nurse.

For a client who needs minimal help:

6. Ask the client to
   a. Grasp the head of the bed with both hands and pull during the move
   or
   b. Raise the upper part of the body on the elbows and push with the hands and forearms during the move
   or

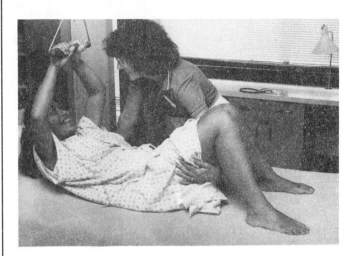

Figure 36–4

   c. Grasp the overhead trapeze with both hands and lift and pull during the move.

   Rationale Client assistance provides additional power to overcome friction during the move. These actions also keep the client's arms partially off the bed surface, reducing friction during movement, and make use of the large muscle groups of the client's arms to increase the force during movement.

7. Face the direction of the movement and assume a broad stance with the foot nearest the bed behind the forward foot and the weight on the forward foot. Incline your trunk forward from the hips. Flex hips, knees, and ankles.

   Rationale Facing the direction of movement prevents twisting of the spine. The broad stance provides balance. Flexing the joints of the lower extremities lowers the center of gravity, increases stability, and ensures use of the large muscle groups in the legs during movement.

8. Place your near arm under the client's thighs and push down on the mattress with the far arm. See Figure 36–4.

   Rationale The near arm supports the heaviest part of the body (the buttocks). The far arm acts as a lever during the move.

9. Tighten your gluteal, abdominal, leg, and arm muscles.

   Rationale Isometric contraction of stabilizing muscles helps to prevent musculoskeletal strain and injury.

10. Rock from the back leg to the front leg and back again; then shift weight to the front leg as the client pushes with the heels and pulls with the arms, moving the client toward the head of the bed.

    Rationale Rocking helps to attain a balanced, smooth motion and to overcome inertia. The nurse's weight shift helps to counteract the client's weight.

11. Elevate the head of the bed. Provide appropriate support devices for the client's new position.

For a client who has limited mobility or strength of the upper extremities:

12. Place the client's arms across the chest.

    Rationale Keeping the client's arms off the bed surface prevents friction during movement.

13. Ask the client to flex the neck during the move.

    Rationale Flexing the neck keeps the head off the bed surface and prevents friction during movement.

14. Position yourself as in step 7.

15. Place one arm under the client's back and shoulders and the other arm under the client's thighs.

    Rationale The placement of the arms distributes the client's weight and supports the heaviest part of the body (the buttocks).

16. Follow steps 9–11 above.

Variation: Two Nurses Using a Hand-Forearm Interlock

Two people are required to move clients who are unable to assist because of their condition or weight. Using the procedure described above, with the second nurse on the opposite side of the bed, the two nurses interlock their forearms under the client's thighs and shoulders and lift the client up in bed. See Figure 36–5.

Variation: Two Nurses Using a Turn Sheet

Two nurses can use a turn sheet to move a client up in the bed. A turn sheet distributes the client's weight more evenly, decreases friction, and exerts a more even force on the client during the move. In addition, it prevents injury of the client's skin, since the friction created between two sheets when one is moved is less than that created by the client's body moving over the sheet.

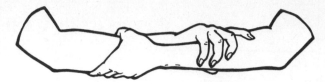

Figure 36–5

A drawsheet or a full sheet folded in half is placed under the client, extending from the shoulders to the thighs.

Each nurse rolls up or fanfolds the turn sheet close to the client's body on either side. The nurses then grasp the sheet close to the shoulders and buttocks of the client. This draws the weight closer to the nurses' base of support, and increases the nurses' balance and stability, permitting a smoother movement. The method described in steps 7, 9, and 10 is then used to move the client up in the bed.

Variation: Pulling a Client Up in Bed

This method emphasizes pulling the client up toward the head of the bed rather than lifting the client. It is designed to create less back strain for the nurse than a method that utilizes lifting. The steps are

17. Follow steps 1–4 as described above.

18. Move the client to the edge of the bed closest to the nurse's body. (Procedure 36–10 describes how to perform this action.)

19. Follow steps 5 and 6 as described above.

    Rationale Client assistance provides additional power to overcome friction during the move.

20. If the client has limited strength of the upper extremities, follow steps 12–13 as described above.

21. Face the foot of the bed, position yourself appropriately, and place both hands together beneath the client's coccyx. The nurse's elbow closest to the client will be beneath the client's upper back. Both elbows should rest on the surface of the bed. Align your body so that it is directly in line with your hands.

    Rationale This placement of the arms, beneath the heaviest part of the client's body, enables the nurse to pull the client directly toward the nurse's center of gravity, preventing spinal twisting. Placement of the nurse's hands focuses and increases the force needed for movement and reduces the friction of the client's body against the bed surface. Resting the elbows on the bed surface prevents inadvertent lifting by the nurse. Pulling rather than pushing can be more comfortable for the client and is safer for the nurse, since she or he retains greater control over the movement.

22. Coordinating your efforts with those of the client, rock backward and shift weight from the forward to the backward foot, pulling the client directly toward you while the client pushes with the heels and pulls with the arms. The hip closest to the bed should slide along the side of the mattress. Your elbows should slide along the bed surface.

    Rationale Rocking backward uses the nurse's body weight to increase the force of movement in the direction of the pull and helps to overcome inertia. Pulling from the client's center of gravity directly toward the nurse's own center of gravity requires less force than lifting and prevents spinal twisting. Keeping elbows on the bed surface also prevents inadvertent lifting by the nurse.

23. Raise the side rail and move to the opposite side of the bed. Move or pull the client as above, and move again to the opposite side of the bed. Move or pull the client back to the center of the bed. Raise the side rail.

    Rationale A raised side rail is essential in preventing the client from falling out of bed.

PROCEDURE 36–10 **Moving a Client to the Side of the Bed in Segments**

This movement is used in preparation for moving the client onto a stretcher, in preparation for turning the client to the lateral (side-lying) position, or when changing the client's bed. Whenever the client is capable of assisting with this movement, he or she should be encouraged to lift the body by holding onto the raised side rail or by using the overhead trapeze. In this movement the nurse's weight is used to counteract the client's weight; the nurse's arms serve as connecting bars between the client and the nurse.

INTERVENTION

1. Assess the client's ability to participate, and explain procedure to client.

2. Stand as close as possible at the side of the bed toward which the client will be moved and opposite the client's chest.

   Rationale Spinal twisting is avoided when the nurse's center of gravity is placed as close as possible to the client's center of gravity and when the direction of movement is squarely faced. This position also lessens the client's fear of falling.

3. Place the client's near arm across his or her chest.

   Rationale Placing the client's arm across the chest avoids friction and resistance to movement and prevents injury to the arm.

4. Incline your trunk forward from the hips. Flex your hips, knees, and ankles. Assume a broad stance, with one foot forward and the weight placed upon this forward foot.

   Rationale The broad stance provides balance. Flexing the joints of the lower extremities lowers the center of gravity, increasing stability, and ensures use of the large muscle groups in the legs during movement.

5. Place your arms and hands with palms facing upward close together beneath the client's scapulae. (If the client cannot support the head during the movement, position your arm nearest the head of the bed so that it cradles the client's head.) Flex your fingers around the client's far shoulder and rest your elbows on the surface of the bed.

   Rationale Placing the arms and hands beneath the heaviest part of the client's upper trunk focuses

and increases the force for movement. Placing the arms close together reduces the friction of the client's body against the bed, making the pull easier. The hand and finger positions increase the force of movement. The elbow position prevents inadvertent lifting by the nurse.

6. Tighten your gluteal, abdominal, leg, and arm muscles.

   Rationale Isometric contraction of stabilizing muscles helps to prevent musculoskeletal strain and injury.

7. Rock backward, shifting your weight from the forward to the backward foot, pulling the client's shoulders directly toward you.

   Rationale Pulling requires less energy than lifting. Rocking backward uses the nurse's body weight to assist with the pull. The enlarged base of support enhances stability. Pulling the client's upper body directly toward the center of gravity requires less force and prevents spinal twisting.

8. To move the client's buttocks, place your arms and hands close together beneath the client's buttocks. Repeat steps 6 and 7, pulling the buttocks to the side of the bed.

9. To move the client's legs and feet, place your hands close together beneath the client's ankles. Repeat steps 6 and 7, pulling the client's legs and feet to the side of the bed.

10. Elevate the side rail next to the client.

    Rationale The side rail is essential to prevent the client from falling off the bed.

Variation: Using a Pull Sheet

A pull sheet beneath the client's trunk and thighs can be used to pull the client to the side of the bed. The nurse rolls up the sheet as close as possible to the client's body and first pulls the client's shoulders, then the buttocks, to the side of the bed. The legs and feet are moved as described in step 9.

PROCEDURE 36–11	**Turning a Client to a Lateral or Prone Position in Bed**

Movement to a lateral (side-lying) position may be necessary when placing a bedpan beneath the client, when changing the client's bed linen, or when repositioning the client.

INTERVENTION

1. Assess the client's ability to participate, and explain procedure to client.

2. Before moving a client to a lateral position, move the client closer to the side of the bed opposite the side the client will face when turned. See Procedure 36–10.

   Rationale This ensures that the client will be positioned safely in the center of the bed after turning.

3. While standing on the side of the bed nearest the client, place the client's near arm across his or her chest. Abduct the client's far shoulder slightly from the side of the body.

   Rationale Placing the one arm forward facilitates the turning motion. Placing the other arm away from the body prevents that arm from being caught beneath the client's body during rolling.

4. Place the client's near ankle and foot across the far ankle and foot. Raise the side rail next to the client before going to the other side of the bed.

   Rationale Placing the near ankle and foot forward facilitates the turning motion. Making these preparations on the side of the bed closest to the client helps the nurse prevent unnecessary reaching. The raised side rail prevents the client who is close to the edge of the mattress from falling out of the bed.

5. Position yourself on the side of the bed toward which the client will turn, directly in line with the client's waistline and as close to the bed as possible.

   Rationale Spinal twisting is avoided when the nurse's center of gravity is placed as close as possible to the client's center of gravity and when the direction of movement is squarely faced.

6. Incline your trunk forward from the hips. Flex your hips, knees, and ankles. Assume a broad stance

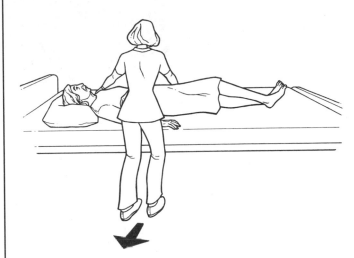

Figure 36–6

with one foot forward and the weight placed upon this forward foot.

Rationale The broad stance provides balance. Flexing the joints of the lower extremities lowers the center of gravity, increasing stability, and ensures use of the large leg muscles during movement.

7. Place one hand on the client's far hip and the other hand on the client's far shoulder. See Figure 36–6.

   Rationale This position of the hands supports the client at the two heaviest parts of the body, providing greater control in movement during the roll.

8. Tighten your gluteal, abdominal, leg, and arm muscles.

   Rationale Isometric contraction of stabilizing muscles helps to prevent musculoskeletal strain and injury.

9. Rock backward, shifting your weight from the forward to the backward foot, and roll the client onto the side to face you. See Figure 36–7.

   Rationale Pulling requires less energy than lifting. Rocking backward uses the nurse's body weight to assist with the pull. The enlarged base of support enhances stability. Pulling the client's body directly toward your own center of gravity requires less force and prevents spinal twisting.

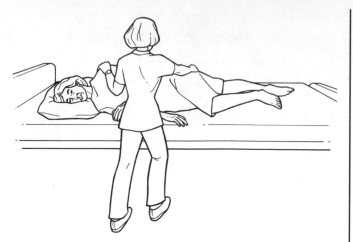

Figure 36−7

Variation: Turning the Client to a Prone Position

To turn a client to the prone position, the nurse follows all of the above steps with two exceptions:

• Instead of abducting the far arm, the client's arm is kept alongside the body for the client to roll over.

Rationale Keeping the arm alongside the body prevents it from being pinned underneath when the client is rolled.

• The client is rolled completely onto the abdomen. It is essential to move the client as close as possible to the bed edge before the turn so that he or she will be lying in the center of the bed after rolling. A client should never be pulled across the bed while in the prone position because doing so can injure the breasts of a woman or the genitals of a man.

PROCEDURE 36–12 **Moving a Client to a Sitting Position on the Edge of the Bed**

The client assumes a sitting position on the edge of the bed before walking, moving to a chair or wheelchair, eating, or performing other activities.

INTERVENTION

1. Assess client's blood pressure, pulse, and respiration. Report signs of hypotension, tachycardia, or tachypnea to nurse in charge *before* beginning procedure. Reschedule activity if indicated.

2. Assist the client to a lateral position facing the nurse. See Procedure 36–11.

3. Raise the head of the bed slowly as high as it will go.

   Rationale This decreases the distance that the client needs to move to sit up on the side of the bed.

4. Position the client's feet and lower legs just to or over the edge of the bed.

   Rationale This enables the client's feet to move easily off the bed during the movement, and the client is aided by gravity into a sitting position.

5. Stand beside the client's hips and face the far corner of the bottom of the bed. Assume a broad stance, placing the foot nearest the client forward. Incline your trunk forward from the hips. Flex your hips, knees, and ankles. See Figure 36–8.

   Rationale The broad stance provides balance. Flexing the joints of the lower extremities lowers the center of gravity, increases stability, and ensures use of the large leg muscles during movement. The nurse avoids twisting of the spine by facing the foot of the bed at the angle in which the movement will occur.

6. Place one arm around the client's shoulders and the other arm beneath both of the client's thighs near the knees. See Figure 36–8.

   Rationale Supporting the client's shoulders prevents the client from falling backward during movement. Supporting the client's thighs reduces friction of the thighs against the bed surface during the move and increases the force of the movement.

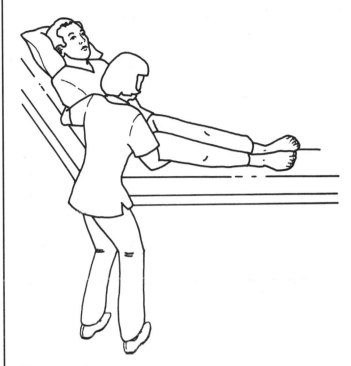

Figure 36–8

7. Tighten your gluteal, abdominal, leg, and arm muscles.

   Rationale Isometric contraction of stabilizing muscles helps to prevent musculoskeletal strain and injury.

8. Lift the client's thighs slightly. Pivot on the balls of your feet while pulling the client's feet and legs off the bed. See Figure 36–9.

   Rationale Raising the thighs off the bed reduces the friction of the client's thighs and the nurse's arm against the bed surface. Pivoting prevents twisting of the nurse's spine. The weight of the client's legs swinging downward increases downward movement of the lower body and helps make the client's upper body vertical.

9. Keep supporting the shoulders and thighs until the client is balanced and comfortable.

   Rationale This movement may cause some clients to feel faint.

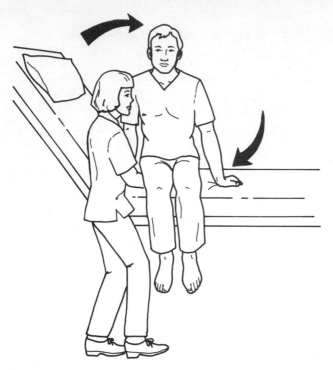

Figure 36–9

Variation: Teaching a Client How to Sit on the Side of the Bed Independently

A client who has had recent abdominal surgery or who is weak may have too much abdominal pain or too little strength to sit straight up in bed. This person can be taught to assume a "dangle" position without assistance. First check agency policy about "dangling." Many cardiovascular units do not allow dangling. If dangling is allowed, instruct the client to

1. Roll to the side and lift the far leg beside the near leg.

2. Grasp the mattress edge with the near arm and push the fist of the upper arm into the mattress.
   or
   If there are upper and lower side rails, grasp the upper side rail and push the fist of the upper arm into the mattress.

3. Push up with both arms (or pull with one arm on the side rail) as the heels and legs slide over the mattress edge.

4. Maintain sitting position by pushing both fists into the mattress behind and to the sides of the buttocks.

PROCEDURE 36–13 **Logrolling a Client**

Logrolling is a procedure used to turn a client whose body must at all times be kept in straight alignment (like a log). An example is the client who has a spinal injury. Considerable care must be taken to prevent additional injury. This procedure requires two nurses or, if the client is large or has a cervical injury, three nurses. For the client who has a cervical injury, one nurse must maintain the client's head and neck alignment.

INTERVENTION

1. Assess the client's injury, and obtain sufficient assistance before beginning procedure.

2. The nurses stand on the same side of the bed and assume a broad stance with one foot ahead of the other.

   Rationale A broad stance enhances balance.

3. Place the client's arms across his or her chest.

   Rationale The client's arms then will not be injured or become trapped under the body.

4. Incline your trunk and flex your hips, knees, and ankles.

   Rationale Flexing these joints ensures use of the large muscle groups in the legs when moving and lowers the center of gravity, enhancing stability.

5. Place your arms under the client as shown in Figure 36–10 or Figure 36–11, depending upon the client's size.

   Rationale Each nurse then has a major weight area of the client centered between the arms.

6. Tighten your gluteal, abdominal, leg, and arm muscles.

   Rationale Isometric contraction of these muscles prepares them for action and prevents injury.

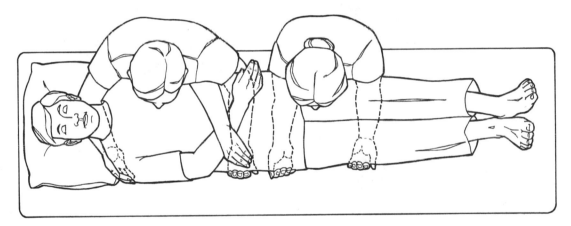

Figure 36–10

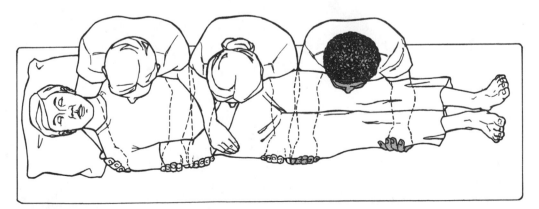

Figure 36–11

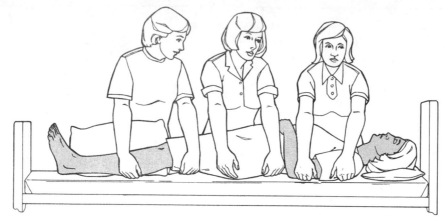

Figure 36-12

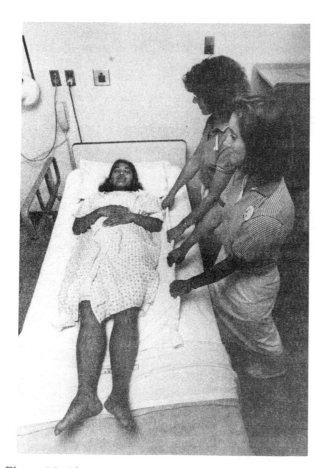

Figure 36-13

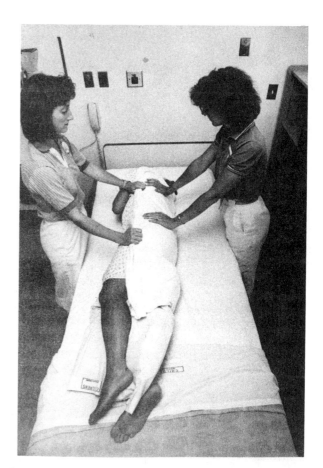

Figure 36-14

7. One nurse counts, "One, two, three, go." Then, at the same time, all nurses pull the client to the side of the bed by rocking backward and shifting weight to the back foot and flexing the knees.

   Rationale Moving the client in unison maintains the client's body alignment.

8. Elevate the side rail on this side of the bed.

   Rationale Elevating the side rail prevents the client from falling while lying so close to the edge of the bed.

9. All nurses move to the other side of the bed.

10. Place a pillow where it will support the client's head after the turn.

    Rationale The pillow prevents lateral flexion of the neck and ensures alignment of the cervical spine.

11. Place one or two pillows between the client's legs to support the upper leg when the client is turned.

    Rationale The pillow between the client's legs prevents adduction of the upper leg and keeps the legs parallel and aligned.

12. All nurses flex the hips, knees, and ankles and assume a broad stance with one foot forward.

13. All nurses reach over the client and place hands as shown in Figure 36–12.

    Rationale This centers a major weight area of the client between each nurse's arms.

14. One nurse counts, "One, two, three, go." Then, at the same time, all nurses roll the client to a lateral position.

15. Place pillows to maintain the client's lateral position.

Variation: Using a Turn Sheet

Logrolling can be facilitated with the use of a turn sheet. The client is first moved to the side of the bed by two nurses who stand on the same side of the bed. Each nurse assumes a broad stance with one foot forward and grasps half of the fanfolded or rolled edge of the turn sheet. On a signal, the nurses pull the client toward them. See Figure 36–13.

Before the client is turned, pillow supports are placed for the head and the legs, as described in steps 10 and 11, to maintain the client's alignment when turning. One nurse then goes to the other side of the bed (farthest from the client) and assumes a stable stance. Reaching over the client, this nurse grasps the far edges of the turn sheet and rolls the client forward. See Figure 36–14. The second nurse (behind the client) helps to turn the client as needed and provides pillow supports to ensure good alignment in the lateral position.

PROCEDURE 36–14 **Transferring a Client to a Chair Using a Mechanical Lifter**

Mechanical lifters are used primarily for clients who cannot help themselves or who are too heavy for others to lift safely. Transfers may be made between the bed and a wheelchair, the bed and the bathtub, and the bed and a stretcher. Various types of mechanical lifters are used to lift and move clients. It is important that nurses be familiar with the model used and the practices that accompany use. Before using the lifter, the nurse ensures that it is in working order and that the hooks, chains, straps, and canvas seat are in good repair. Most agencies recommend that two nurses operate a lifter. Agency policy should be checked in this regard.

Before lifting the client, the nurse explains the procedure and demonstrates the lifter. Some clients are afraid of being lifted and will be reassured by a demonstration.

The lifter may have a one-piece or two-piece canvas seat. The one-piece seat stretches from the client's head to the knees. The two-piece seat has one canvas strap to support the client's buttocks and thighs and a second strap to support the back, extending up to the axillae.

EQUIPMENT

• A mechanical lifter

• A chair

INTERVENTION

1. Assess client for signs of cardio-respiratory distress before beginning. Check with nurse in charge if distress noted.

2. Place the chair that is to receive the client beside the bed. Allow room for the lifter and the client to clear the bed and the chair.

3. Lock the wheels, if a chair with wheels is used.
   Rationale This prevents the chair from moving under the client.

4. Put the canvas seat or straps exactly in place under the client. See Figure 36–15.
   Rationale Correct placement permits the client to be lifted evenly, with minimal shifting.

5. Wheel the lifter into position at a right angle to the side of the bed, with the footbars under the bed. Lock the wheels of the lifter and the bed.

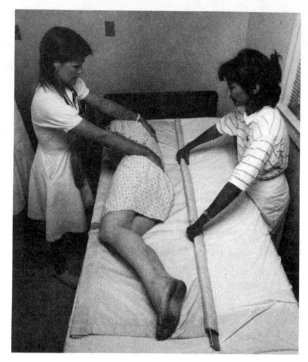

Figure 36–15

6. Ask the client to remove eyeglasses, and put them in a safe place.
   Rationale The client should not wear glasses because the swivel bar may come close to the face.

7. Attach the lifter straps or hooks to the corresponding openings in the canvas seat. Check that the hooks are correctly placed and that matching straps or chains are of equal length.

8. To lift the client:
   a. *Nurse 1:* Close the pressure valve, and gradually pump up the lift until the client is above the bed surface.
      Rationale Gradual elevation of the lift is less frightening to the client than a rapid rise.
   b. *Nurse 2:* Assume a broad stance and tighten your abdominal and pelvic muscles. Guide the client with your hands as the client is lifted.
      Rationale The nurse prepares to hold the client and provide control during the movement.

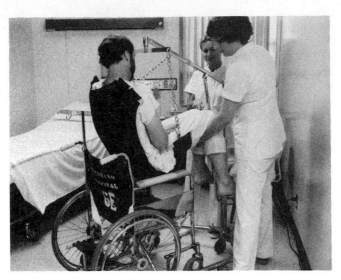

Figure 36—16

9. To move the client:
   a. *Nurse 1:* With the pressure valve securely closed, slowly roll the lifter until the client is over the chair.

b. *Nurse 2:* Guide movement by hand until the client is directly over the chair. See Figure 36—16.

   Rationale Slow movement decreases swaying and is less frightening. Guidance also decreases swaying and gives a sense of security.

10. To lower the client into the chair;
    a. *Nurse 1:* Release the pressure valve very gradually.
    b. *Nurse 2:* Guide the client into the chair.

    Rationale Gradual release lowers the client slowly and is less frightening than a quick descent.

11. Remove the hooks from the canvas seat. Leave the seat in place.

    Rationale The seat is left in place in preparation for the lift back to bed.

12. Align the client appropriately in a sitting position. Give the client his or her glasses if appropriate.

CASTS

CAST MATERIALS

In addition to the traditional plaster of paris cast material, several synthetic materials are now available: polyester and cotton, fiberglass, and thermoplastics. See Table 36–1. Advantages of the synthetic casts compared to plaster of paris casts include:

1. They dry and set quickly, so they can bear weight within a short period of time.

2. They are lightweight, so they restrict mobility less.

3. They are less bulky, so regular clothing can be worn over them.

4. They are less likely to become indented while drying.

5. They do not crumble at the edges, and any rough cast edges can be smoothed with a nail file or emery board.

6. They can be immersed in water if the physician permits and if a nonabsorbent synthetic lining such as polypropylene stockinette and polyester padding is used. (Plaster of paris is weakened by moisture and must be kept dry at all times.) Synthetic casts must be thoroughly dried, however (see disadvantage 4, later).

7. They are easily kept clean with water and small amounts of a mild, nonirritating soap.

Table 36–1
Characteristics of Cast Materials

Characteristics	Plaster of paris	Synthetics		
		Polyester and cotton (eg, Cutter Cast)	Fiberglass; water-activated (eg, Scotchcast, Delta-lite) or light-cured (eg, Lightcast II)	Thermoplastic (eg, Hexcelite)
Description	Open-weave cotton rolls or strips saturated with powdered calcium sulfate crystals (gypsum)	Open-weave polyester and cotton tape permeated with water-activated polyurethane resin	Open-weave fiberglass tape impregnated with water-activated polyurethane resin (Scotchcast) or photo-sensitive polyurethane resin (Lightcast II)	Knitted thermoplastic polyester fabric in rigid rolls
Application	Applied after being soaked in tepid water for a few seconds until bubbling stops	Applied after being soaked in cool water, 26 C (80 F)	Applied after being soaked in tepid water (Scotchcast); applied with silicone type hand cream to keep it from sticking (Lightcast II)	Applied after being heated in water at 76 to 82 C (170 to 180 F) for 3 to 4 minutes to make the rolls soft and pliable
Setting time and weight-bearing restrictions	Dries in 48 hours, no weight bearing allowed until dry	Sets in 7 minutes, weight bearing allowed in 15 minutes	Sets in 15 minutes, weight bearing allowed in 30 minutes (Scotchcast); sets after being exposed for 3 minutes to a special ultraviolet lamp, weight bearing allowed immediately (Lightcast II)	Sets in 5 minutes, weight bearing allowed in 20 minutes

SOURCE: PL Lane, MM Lee: New synthetic casts: What nurses need to know. *Orthop Nurs* (November/December) 1982; 1(6); 13–20.

8. Foreign particles that gain entrance to the cast can be flushed out with water.

Disadvantages of the synthetic casts include:

1. They are more expensive (3 to 8 times more than plaster of paris material).

2. They cannot be molded as readily as plaster of paris to fit limb contours, so they are not as effective for immobilizing severely displaced fractures or fractures that produce excessive edema.

3. Their surfaces are rougher than plaster of paris, so they can snag clothes, scratch furniture, and abrade the skin on the opposite extremity.

4. There is an increased chance of skin maceration if proper drying procedures are not followed. When the cast becomes wet, excess water must be blotted with a towel, and a blow dryer must be used, on the cool or warm setting, over the entire cast until it is completely dry.

5. Vigorous activity can misalign the fracture or break the cast.

TYPES OF CASTS

The following are types of casts for the arm, leg, and trunk of the body:

1. The hanging arm cast extends from the axilla to the fingers of the hand, usually allowing for elbow flexion. See Figure 36–17, A. It immobilizes the wrist, the humerus, the radius, and the ulna.

2. The short arm cast extends from below the elbow to the fingers. See Figure 36–17, B. It immobilizes the wrist, the radius, and the ulna.

3. The shoulder spica cast extends around the chest and the entire arm to the fingers. The arm is usually abducted to immobilize the shoulder bones, eg, the clavicle. See Figure 36–17, C.

4. The long or full leg cast extends from above the knee to the toes. See Figure 36–17, D.

5. The short leg cast begins just below the knee and extends to the toes. See Figure 36–17, E.

6. The hip spica cast begins at waist level or above. It immobilizes the hip joint and the femur, extends down one entire leg, and may cover all or part of the second leg. A single spica covers one leg only. See Figure 36–17, F. A one-and-one-half hip spica covers the second leg to the knee. See Figure 36–17, G. A double hip spica covers both legs to the toes.

7. The body cast extends from the axillae to encompass the entire trunk. It is often used to immobilize the spine.

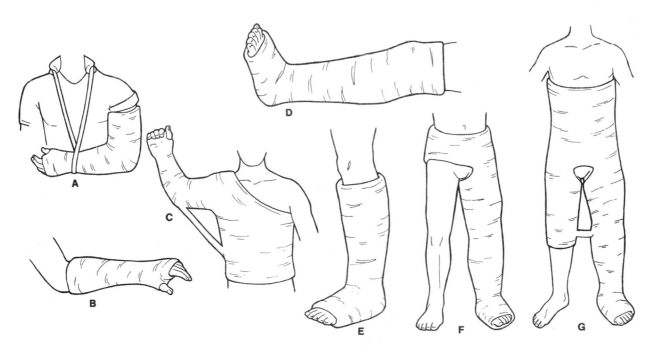

Figure 36–17
Types of cylindrical casts: **A**, hanging arm cast; **B**, short arm cast; **C**, shoulder spica; **D**, long leg cast; **E**, short leg cast; **F**, single hip spica; **G**, one-and-one-half hip spica.

PROCEDURE 36–15 **Client Care Immediately After Cast Application**

Nursing interventions immediately after cast application include

- Neurovascular assessment of affected limbs
- Supporting and handling the cast appropriately until it sets
- Actions to reduce swelling
- Actions to promote drying of the cast
- Monitoring any drainage or bleeding
- Assessing pain and signs of pressure beneath the cast
- Documenting assessments and interventions

EQUIPMENT

- Soft, pliable pillows

INTERVENTION

Neurovascular Assessment

1. Assess the toes and fingers for nerve or circulatory impairments every 30 minutes for several hours following application and then every 3 hours for the first 24–48 hours or until all signs and symptoms of impairment are negative. Rapid swelling under a cast can cause neurovascular problems necessitating frequent neurovascular assessments by the nurse.

Supporting and Handling the Cast

2. Immediately after the cast is applied, place it on pillows. Avoid using plastic or rubber pillows.

   Rationale The pillows provide even pressure and support the curves of the cast and promote venous blood return, thereby decreasing the possibility of swelling. Plastic or rubber pillows do not allow the heat of a drying cast to dissipate and so cause discomfort.

3. Until a cast has set or hardened (10–20 minutes), support the cast in the palms of your hands rather than with the fingertips. Some authorities advocate that you extend your fingers so that your fingertips do not touch the plaster. See Figure 36–18. When the cast is set, continue to handle the cast

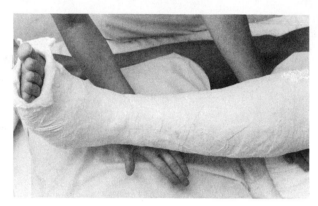

Figure 36–18

in your palms, but you may then wrap your fingers around the contour of the cast.

Rationale Fingertip pressure can cause dents in unset plaster and subsequent skin pressure areas.

Reducing Swelling

4. Control swelling by elevating arms or legs on pillows or, for a leg fracture, by elevating the foot of the bed. Immediately after injury and surgery, elevate the limb well above the level of the client's heart. Generally, three pillows are needed to achieve high elevation of a leg. As circulation improves and healing progresses, the elevation can be gradually reduced to two pillows (moderate elevation) and then to one pillow (low elevation).

   Rationale Swelling can cause neurovascular impairment.

5. Report excessive swelling and indications of neurovascular impairment to the physician or nurse in charge. The physician may bivalve a cast if it appears to be too tight. Bivalving a cast is cutting the cast and the underlying padding on each side, thus making two separate shells. See Figure 36–19, *A*. This relieves the pressure of the cast but still provides support. Bivalved casts are usually fastened in place with Velcro straps, buckled webbing straps, or elastic bandages. See Figure 36-19, *B*.

6. Apply ice packs to control perineal edema associated with a hip spica cast. Although ice packs are a less effective method of control, elevation of the area is obviously difficult.

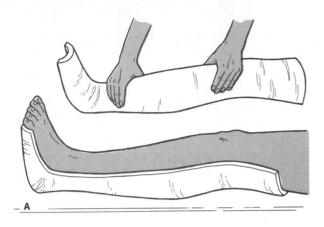

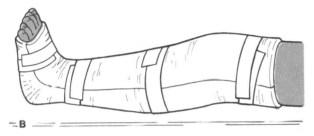

Figure 36–19

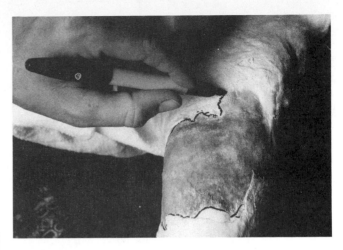

Figure 36–20

Drying the Cast

Extremity plaster of paris casts usually take 24–48 hours to dry completely; spica or body casts require 48–72 hours. Drying time depends on the temperature, humidity, size of the cast, and method used for drying. The cast is dry when it no longer feels damp. A dry cast feels dry and looks white and shiny and is odorless, hard, and resonant when tapped. Fiberglass casts usually require less drying time and are available in a variety of colors.

7. Expose the cast to the circulating air. Place sheets and blankets only over areas that do not have the cast.

8. Check agency policy about the recommended turning frequency for clients with different kinds of casts.

   Rationale Frequent turning promotes even drying of the cast.

9. Turn the client with an extremity cast or body spica every 2–4 hours. See Procedure 36–16, step 14.

10. Use regular pillows.

    Rationale Plastic or rubber pillows hinder drying and do not allow the heat of a drying cast to dissipate.

11. Avoid the use of artificial means to facilitate drying. These means include fans, hair driers, infrared lamps, and electric heaters.

    Rationale Artificial methods dry the outer surface of the cast while the inner portion remains soft and spongy. Such a cast cracks readily at points of strain. Natural methods dry the cast evenly.

Monitoring Drainage

12. If an open reduction has been done or if the injury was a compound fracture, bleeding may occur, and the cast may become stained with blood.

    a. Monitor such drainage for 24–72 hours after surgery or injury, or longer if necessary.

    b. Outline the stained area with a pen every 8 hours or at the change of shift, and note the time and date, so that any further bleeding can be determined. See Figure 36–20.

Assessing Pain and Pressure Areas

13. Never ignore any complaints of pain, burning, or pressure. If a client is unable to communicate, be alert to changes in temperament, restlessness, or fussiness.

14. Determine particularly whether the pain is persistent and if it occurs over a bony prominence or joint. See Table 36–2 for common pressure points associated with various casts.

15. Give pain medications selectively.

    Rationale Pain medication can mask symptoms.

16. Do not disregard the cessation of persistent pain or discomfort complaints.

Table 36-2
Common Cast Pressure Areas

Type of cast	Common pressure areas
Short arm cast	Radial styloid
	Ulnar styloid
	Joint at base of thumb
Hanging arm cast	Radial styloid
	Ulnar styloid
	Olecranon
	Lateral epicondyle
Short leg cast	Heel
	Achilles tendon
	Malleolus
Long leg cast	Heel
	Achilles tendon
	Malleolus
	Popliteal artery behind knee
	Peroneal nerve at side of knee
Hip spica	As above for long leg cast
	Sacrum
	Iliac crests

Rationale Cessation of complaints can indicate a skin slough. When a skin slough occurs superficial skin sensation is lost and the client no longer feels pain.

17. When a pressure area under the cast is suspected the physician may either bivalve the cast so that all of the skin beneath the cast can be inspected or cut a window in the cast over only the area of concern. When a cast is windowed

   a. Retain the piece (cast and padding) that was cut out. Some physicians order that it be taped back if there is no skin problem present but that it be left out if there is a pressure area present.

   Rationale Putting back the piece prevents window edema, which occurs when skin pressure at the window is not equal to that from the remainder of the cast.

   b. Inspect the skin under the window at scheduled intervals.

18. Document each assessment (whether or not there are problems) and implementation. Examples of documentation include: "Toes warm to touch, color pink," or "Toes cold, pale, and edematous"; "Blanching sign satisfactory," or "Slow return of blood from blanching sign"; "Moves toes readily; states no numbness or tingling; states leg painful," or "C/o numbness and tingling in toes; movement decreased." Record specific nerve function assessments such as "Able to hyperextend R thumb"; "Sensation felt at web space between R thumb and index finger."

PROCEDURE 36–16 **Continuing Care for Clients with Casts**

Continuing care for clients with casts involves (a) providing meticulous skin care, (b) keeping the cast clean and dry, (c) turning and positioning the client appropriately, (d) encouraging active exercise, and (e) teaching cast care.

EQUIPMENT

For skin care:

- Rubbing alcohol
- Mineral, olive, or baby oil to apply to the skin after cast removal

For covering rough cast edges:

- Adhesive tape 2.5 cm (1 in.) wide
- Scissors

For keeping the cast clean and dry:

- A damp washcloth for plaster of paris casts
- Warm water and a mild soap for synthetic casts

For comfort:

- Pillows
- A slipper (fracture) pan

INTERVENTION

1. Obtain baseline assessment data.

Skin Care

The skin near and under the cast edges is inspected whenever neurovascular assessments are made and/or whenever the client is turned. To prevent skin irritation at the edges of a cast, implement the following measures:

2. Wash crumbs of plaster from the skin with a damp cloth and feel along the cast edges to check for rough edges or areas that press into the client's skin. It may be necessary to use a duckbilled cast bender to bend cast edges that may irritate the skin. See Figure 36–21. Excessive bending or

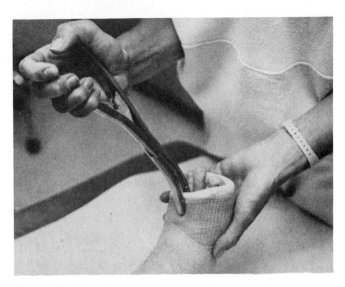

Figure 36–21

trimming of the cast should not be done without a physician's order.

Rationale As a plaster of paris cast dries, small bits of plaster frequently break off from its rough edges. If they fall inside the cast, they can cause discomfort and irritation.

3. Cover any rough edges of the cast when it is dry. If stockinette has not been used to line the cast, "petal" the edges with small strips of adhesive tape as follows (see Figure 36–22):

   a. Cut several strips of 2.5 cm (1 in.) nonwaterproof adhesive, 5–7.5 cm (2–3 in.) long. Then curve all corners of each strip. See Figure 36–23.

   Rationale Square or pointed ends tend to curl. Nonwaterproof adhesive is more adherent.

   b. Insert one end of each strip as far as possible inside the cast, and bring the other end out over the cast edge. See Figure 36–24.

   c. Press the petals firmly against the plaster. See Figure 36–25.

   d. Overlap successive petals slightly.

4. Check the cast daily for a foul odor.

   Rationale This kind of odor may indicate skin excoriation from pressure or an infected area beneath the cast.

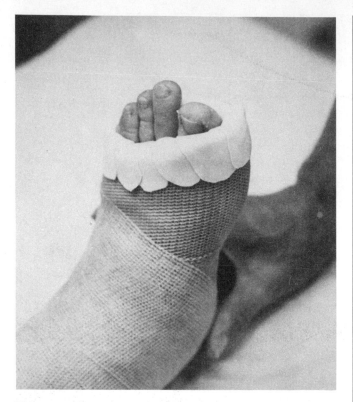

Figure 36—22

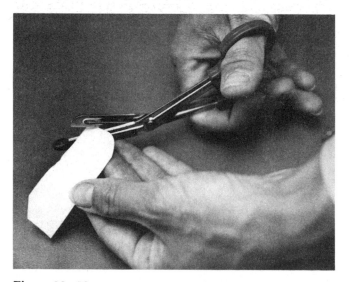

Figure 36—23

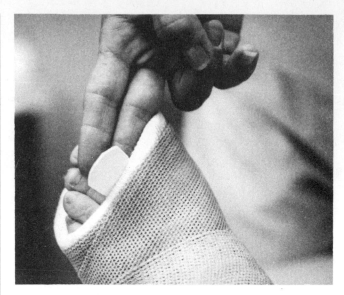

Figure 36—24

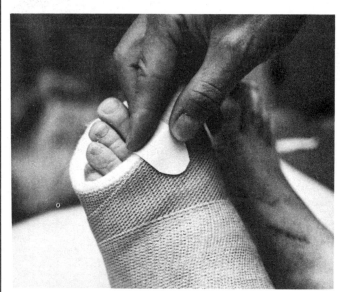

Figure 36—25

5. Provide skin care, using alcohol, to all areas vulnerable to pressure and breakdown at least every 4 hours. For clients with sensitive skin or potential skin problems, provide care every 2 hours during the day and every 3 hours at night.

   Rationale Alcohol cleans and toughens the skin and evaporates without making the cast soggy.

   a. Reach under the cast edges as far as possible and massage the area.

   b. Also provide skin care over all bony prominences not under the cast, eg, the sacrum, heels, ankles, wrists, elbows, and feet.

   Rationale These are potential pressure areas while the client is confined to bed.

6. Itching is a common problem.

   a. Discourage the person from using long sharp objects to scratch under the cast.

   Rationale These objects can break the skin and cause an infection, since bacteria flourish in the warm, dark, moist environment under the cast.

b. Suggest that the client tap the cast or, at home, use a hair drier on cool, a vacuum cleaner on reverse, or an ice bag over the outside of the itching area.

Rationale These are safer ways to resolve itching and less irritating to the skin.

7. When healing is complete and the cast is removed, the underlying skin is usually dry, flaky, and encrusted, since layers of dead skin have accumulated. Remove this debris gently and gradually.

a. Apply oil (eg, mineral, olive, or baby oil).

b. Soak the skin in warm water and dry it.

c. Caution the client not to rub the area too vigorously.

Rationale Vigorous rubbing can cause bleeding or excoriation.

d. Repeat steps a and b for several days.

Rationale Gradual removal of skin exudate avoids skin irritation.

Keeping the Cast Clean and Dry

8. *Plaster of paris casts:* Because these casts are porous and will absorb water or urine, every effort is made to keep them dry. Casts that become wet soften, and their function is impaired; thus, tub baths and showers are contraindicated. Casts that become soiled with feces develop an unremovable odor. Elimination presents a particular problem for people with long leg, body, and hip spica casts. There is no effective way to keep a plaster of paris cast clean other than wiping it with a damp cloth. Before a client is discharged, a cast may be cleaned by applying more wet plaster over the soiled area. The best approach is to prevent soils and stains, especially those from food spills, urine, and feces.

a. Place a bib or towel over a body cast to catch spills. If a spill does wet the cast, allow the area to air dry.

b. Use a slipper (fracture) bedpan for people with long leg, hip spica, or body casts.

Rationale The flat end placed correctly under the client's buttocks lessens the chance of spillage and minimizes the amount of lifting required by the client and/or nurse.

c. Before placing the client on the bedpan, tuck plastic or other waterproof material around the top of a long leg cast or in around the perineal cutout. For a perineal cutout, funnel one end of the plastic into the bedpan.

d. Remove the plastic when elimination is completed.

Rationale If left in place, waterproof material makes the cast edge airtight and prevents evaporation of perspiration, which is irritating to the skin.

e. For people with long leg casts, keep the cast supported on pillows while the client is on the bedpan.

Rationale If the cast dangles, urine may run down the cast.

f. For clients with hip spica casts, support both extremities and the back on pillows so that they are as high as the buttocks.

Rationale This prevents urine from running back into the cast.

g. When removing the bedpan, hold it securely while the client is turning or lifting the buttocks.

Rationale This prevents dripping and spilling.

h. After removing the bedpan, thoroughly clean and dry the perineal area.

9. *Synthetic casts:* Synthetic casts can be cleaned readily and may, with the physician's permission, be immersed in water if polypropylene stockinette and padding were applied.

a. Wash the soiled area with warm water and a mild soap.

b. Thoroughly rinse the soap from the cast.

c. Dry thoroughly to prevent skin maceration and ulceration under the cast.

d. If the cast is immersed in water, the cast and underlying padding and stockinette must be dried thoroughly. First blot excess water from the cast with a towel. Then use a handheld blow drier on the cool or warm setting, directing the air stream in a sweeping motion over the exterior of the cast for about 1 hour or until the client no longer feels a cold clammy sensation like that produced by a wet bathing suit.

Rationale This drying procedure is essential to prevent skin maceration and ulceration.

Turning and Positioning Clients

Correct body alignment, turning, and positioning are absolutely necessary to prevent the formation of pressure areas.

10. Place pillows in such a way that
    a. Body parts press against the cast edges as little as possible.
    b. Toes, heels, elbows, etc, are protected from pressure against the bed surface.
    c. Body alignment is maintained.

11. Plan and implement a turning schedule incorporating all possible positions. Generally, clients can be placed in lateral, prone, and supine positions unless surgical procedures or other factors contraindicate them. A trapeze should be attached to the Balkan frame to enable the client to assist with moving.
    Rationale Repositioning prevents pressure areas.

12. Turn people with large casts or those unable to turn themselves at least once every 4 hours. If the person is at risk for skin breakdown, turn every 1–3 hours as needed.

13. When turning the client in a long leg cast to the unaffected side, place a pillow between the legs to support the cast.

14. At least three persons are needed to turn a person in a damp hip spica cast. When the cast is dry the individual can usually turn with the assistance of one nurse. To turn a client from the supine to prone position, follow these steps:
    a. Remove the support pillows only when an assistant is supporting the cast.
    b. Move the client to one side of the bed.
    c. Ask the client to place the arms above the head or along the sides.
    d. Have two assistants go to the other side of the bed while you remain to provide security for the person who is at the edge of the bed.
    e. Place pillows along the bed surface to receive the cast when the client turns.
    f. Roll the client toward the two assistants onto the pillows.
    g. Adjust the pillows as needed so that they provide proper support and comfort, and prevent pressure areas.

Exercise

15. Unless contraindicated, encourage active ROM exercises for all joints on the unaffected extremities, as well as on the joints proximal and distal to the cast. If active exercises are contraindicated, implement active-assistive or passive exercises, depending on the client's abilities and disabilities.

Rationale Exercise prevents joint stiffness and muscle atrophy.

16. Encourage the client to move toes and/or fingers of the casted extremity as frequently as possible.
    Rationale Moving these extremities enhances peripheral circulation and decreases swelling and pain.

17. With the physician's approval, teach isometric (muscle-setting) exercises.
    Rationale Isometric exercises will minimize muscle atrophy in the affected limb.
    a. Teach the isometric exercises on the client's unaffected limb before the person applies them to the affected limb.
    b. Demonstrate muscle palpation while the client is carrying out the exercise.
    Rationale Palpation enables the person to feel the changes that occur with muscle contraction and relaxation.

Meeting the Client's Learning Needs

Common learning needs include cast care, ways to move effectively with casts, and instructions before discharge.

18. Teach parents of young children ways to prevent the child from placing small items under the cast. One approach is to avoid giving the child small play items such as marbles, pencils, or crayons. Parents also need to ensure that the top of a body cast is covered during meals so that food does not fall inside the cast.

19. Teach people immobilized in bed with large body casts ways to turn and to move safely by using a trapeze, the side rails, etc.

20. Instruct clients with leg casts about ways to walk effectively with crutches.

21. Instruct people with arm casts how to apply slings.

22. Instruct all clients about isometric exercises for extremities in a cast, to prevent muscle atrophy. See the discussion in step 17.

23. Before discharge from the hospital, instruct the client to
    a. Observe for indications of nerve or circulatory impairment, such as extreme coldness or blueness of toes or fingers; extreme continuous swelling of casted toes or fingers; numbness or tingling ("pins and needles" sensation) in casted toes or fingers; continuous

complaints of pain; or inability to move the toes or fingers.

b. Keep the cast dry.

c. Avoid strenuous activity and follow medical advice about exercises.

d. Elevate the arm or leg frequently to prevent dependent edema.

e. Move the toes or fingers frequently.

f. Observe the skin around the cast edges frequently, and keep it clean and dry.

g. Report any increase in pain; unexplained fever; foul odor from within the cast; decreased circulation; numbness; inability to move the fingers or toes; or a weakened, cracked, loose, or tight cast.

24. Document assessments and nursing implementations on the appropriate records.

TRACTION CARE

Traction, like a cast, is a device by which a part of the body is immobilized. But unlike a cast, traction involves a pulling force that is applied to a part of the body, while a second force, called *countertraction*, pulls in the opposite direction. The pulling force of traction is provided through a system of pulleys, ropes, and weights attached to the client; the countertraction is often supplied by the client's body. In balanced traction, the amount of force in the traction is equal to the amount of force in the countertraction. A *suspension* is a mechanism that suspends a body part by using traction equipment, but it does not involve a pulling force. However, traction may be added to a suspension.

In *straight* or *running traction*, the traction force is pulled against the long axis of the body, and the countertraction is supplied by the client's body. In a *suspension* or in a *balanced traction*, the affected part is supported by a sling, hammock, or ring splint, and countertraction is supplied partly by the body and partly by a system of weights attached to an overhead frame with pulleys and ropes.

Clients who have traction are often confined to bed for weeks or even months. Nursing therefore involves activities of daily living, maintenance of the traction, and the prevention of problems such as pressure sores.

PURPOSES OF TRACTION

1. To reduce and/or immobilize a fracture for healing. To *reduce* a fracture is to realign the bones.
2. To correct, reduce, or prevent deformities.
3. Prior to surgery, eg, hip replacement, to provide more space within the hip joint.
4. To decrease muscle spasm before a fracture is reduced.
5. To treat inflammatory conditions by immobilizing a joint, eg, for arthritis or tuberculosis of a joint.

TYPES OF TRACTION

There are four types of traction: manual, skin, skeletal, and encircling.

1. *Manual traction* is applied by the hands, ie, the nurse holds the limb while exerting pulling force. It is a temporary measure used while skin traction is being prepared, eg, when a cast is being applied; or in an emergency, eg, when a traction rope breaks.
2. *Skin traction* is a pulling force applied to the skin and soft tissues through the use of tape or traction straps and a system of ropes, pulleys, and weights. The traction strap is often made of vented foam rubber or cloth, and it may have either an adhesive or nonadhesive backing. Adhesive skin traction is used only for continuous traction. Nonadhesive skin traction is used intermittently; it can easily be removed and applied.
3. *Skeletal traction* is applied by inserting metal pins or wires directly into or through a bone. The metal device is then attached to a system of ropes, pulleys, and weights by means of a metal frame attached to the bed.
4. *Encircling traction* is often considered a type of skin traction. A halter or sling is placed around a body part and attached by means of a rope and pulley to a weight that pulls in a straight line. Examples of encircling traction are cervical head halter traction and pelvic traction.

Traction can be either continuous or intermittent. Continuous traction (skeletal or skin) should be applied and released by a physician, and a physician should be responsible for handling the affected part when it is not in traction. Intermittent traction (nonadhesive skin traction), on the other hand, can be applied and released by nursing personnel with the appropriate physician's order.

TRACTION EQUIPMENT

The following equipment is required for all traction:

1. An overhead frame. This frame is attached to the hospital bed and provides a means for attachment of the traction apparatus (see Figure 36–26). There are a number of kinds of overhead frames, which attach to the bed in different ways; each frame, however, has at least two upright bars and one overhead bar.
2. A trapeze. Attached to the overhead frame, the trapeze can be used by the client for moving in bed, unless contraindicated by the client's condition.
3. A firm mattress. To maintain body alignment and the efficiency of the traction, a firm mattress is essential. Some beds are manufactured with a solid

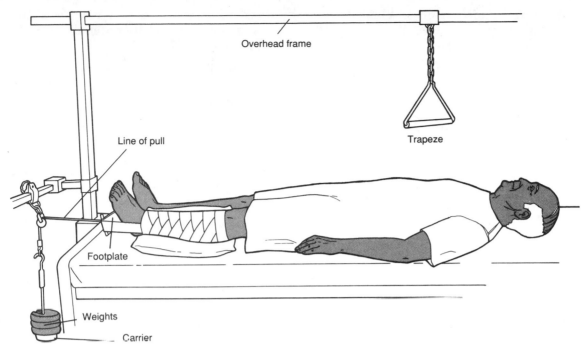

Figure 36–26
Unilateral Buck's extension traction.

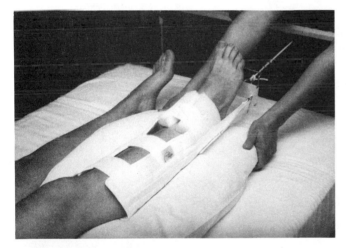

Figure 36–27
A commercially made Buck's boot.

bottom instead of springs, to provide firm support. If a firm bed is not available, a bed board can be used to provide the needed support.

SPECIFIC TRACTIONS

Specific tractions that nurses may see in a hospital include the following.

1. *Buck's extension.* This is a simple traction that can be applied to one leg (unilateral) or both legs (bilateral). See Figure 36–26. It is a skin traction and may use either adhesive or nonadhesive tape. Sometimes commercially made foam rubber boot-type splints with self-adhering straps are used (see Figure 26–27).

2. *Russell traction.* This is a skin traction (adhesive or nonadhesive) applied to one or both legs. A sling is used under the knee to suspend the limb. See Figure 36–28. The pull on the limb is both vertical through the sling and horizontal through the footplate. The degree of flexion of the knee depends on the angle needed as determined by the physician. The placement of the overhead pulley and the pulley on the foot of the bed will vary. The latter may be raised so that it is in line with the pulley on the footplate. The foot of the bed may or may not be elevated for countertraction. A pillow may or may not be ordered to support the lower leg. A variation of Russell traction is called *Split Russell.* In this traction, the weights are applied to the knee and the foot using separate cords; the cord from the sling usually runs to the overhead frame and then to the head of the bed.

3. *Thomas leg splint and Pearson attachment.* The Thomas leg splint consists of a full ring or a half ring around the thigh with two rods on either side of the leg. A sling is attached to the rods of the splint. A foam rubber pad or sheepskinlike material is used in some agencies for the sling. The Pearson attachment is a sling construction that supports the lower leg off the bed and permits the knee to be flexed. Countertraction is supplied mostly by the body's weight. This is a suspension that can be used with skin and/or skeletal traction. See Figure 36–29 for a balanced suspension using a Thomas splint and Pearson attachment in conjunction with both skin and skeletal traction.

4. *Pelvic belt traction.* Pelvic belts (girdles) provide traction to the client's lower back. See Figure 36–30. The belts in common use today are disposable and adjustable, with self-adhering straps. The belt is fitted directly on the skin over the iliac crests (ie, the top margin is at the level of the umbilicus) and fastened over the abdomen. The straps, which attach to the pulley and weight system, may be attached either at the client's sides, so that the pull of the traction is toward the foot of the bed, or at the back (under the client), so that the traction pull is downward and toward the foot of the bed. Countertraction is provided by elevating the foot of the

bed. This type of traction requires a supine position, unless otherwise ordered, and is frequently intermittent.

5. *Cervical head halter traction.* The cervical head halter provides skin (encircling) traction on the cervical spine. See Figure 36–31. The head halter is attached to a spread bar wide enough to prevent the halter from pressing on the client's ears, jaws, or sides of the head. Countertraction from the

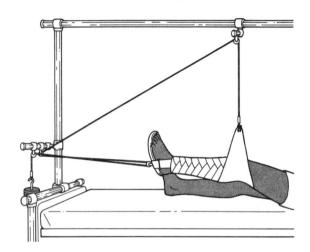

Figure 36–28
Russell traction.

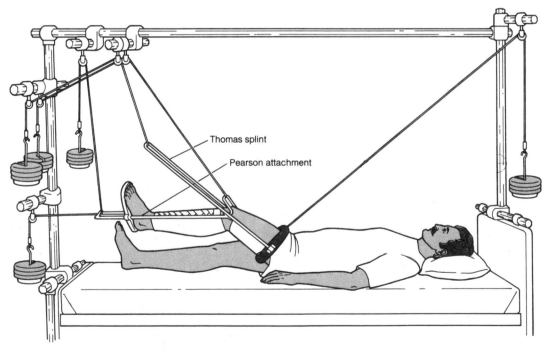

Figure 36–29
Balanced suspension with Thomas leg splint and Pearson attachment.

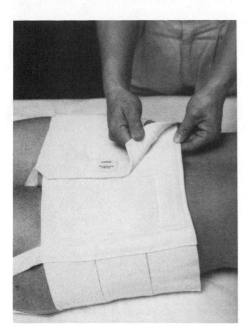

Figure 36–30
Pelvic belt.

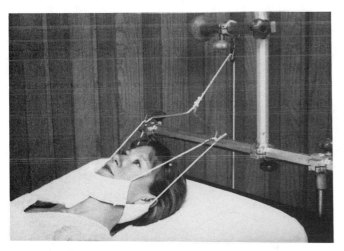

Figure 36–31
Cervical head halter traction.

client's body weight is provided by elevating the head of the bed. Head halter traction may be applied intermittently or continuously. If traction is required for long periods of time, however, skeletal traction is applied.

6. *Halo-thoracic vest traction.* The halo-thoracic traction consists of a circular metal band (tiara or halo) that is fixed to the head by four pins (two anterior and two posterior). See Figure 36–32. These pins penetrate the skull only a fraction of an inch. The halo clears the head by about 1½ cm

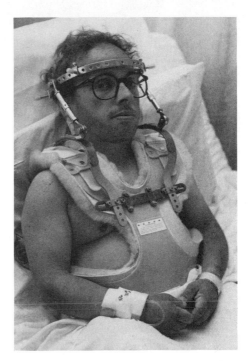

Figure 36–32
Halo-thoracic vest traction.

(½ in.). Attached to the halo are metal rods that are in turn attached to either a plaster cast or plastic vest worn on the client's trunk. Some vests extend to the client's pelvic girdle. The vest, which is well padded with sheepskin, supports and suspends the weight of the entire apparatus around the client's chest.

Halo traction is applied under local anesthetic. It provides firm stabilization of the thoracic spine. Traction to the thoracic spine is achieved by adjusting the nuts and bolts that attach the metal bars to the halo apparatus. By increasing or decreasing the distance between the halo and the vest, traction is increased or decreased. The advantage of this traction over other types of head and neck traction is that it allows the client to sit, stand, and walk, thus decreasing the respiratory, circulatory, and muscular problems associated with prolonged immobility.

7. *Side-arm traction.* Side-arm traction may be skeletal or skin traction, depending on the site of the fracture, the presence of other injuries, and the physician's choice. The traction pull is outward from the upper arm and upward from the forearm. Countertraction is provided by the positioning of the body; for example, a folded blanket placed under the mattress on the side of the traction frame will augment countertraction.

PROCEDURE 36–17 **Applying Nonadhesive Skin Traction**

Nonadhesive skin traction does not cause the skin irritations that are associated with adhesive tape. Furthermore, with the appropriate order, it can be released and applied by nurses. This type of traction is applied to an extremity.

EQUIPMENT

- Doughnut of stockinette to protect the malleoli of the ankle.

- Nonadhesive traction straps.

- 2-in. or 3-in. elastic bandage, depending on the circumference of the extremity.

- Adhesive tape to secure the elastic bandage.

- Footplate or block or spreader bar (see figures 36–26 and 36–27) wide enough to prevent the traction straps from irritating the skin over the sides of the foot and ankle. These come equipped with an attachment for the rope.

- Rope, weight hanger, and weights.

INTERVENTION

1. Assess the skin on the affected extremity.

2. Wash and dry the extremity, ie, the foot and leg.

3. Apply a piece of rolled stockinette over the foot to a point just above the malleoli of the ankle.
   Rationale This protects the skin over these bony prominences from abrasion and pressure from the traction tape.

4. Place the nonadhesive traction strap down the inner aspect of the leg, around the foot, and up the lateral aspect of the leg, leaving the tape slack around the foot.
   Rationale The slack of the tape will be taken up by the spreader bar or footplate.

5. Secure an elastic bandage over the strap, starting just above the ankle, using spiral-reverse or modified figure-eight turns. (See Figure 36–33).
   Rationale Starting just above the ankle avoids placing pressure on the Achilles tendon, and a spiral-reverse or modified figure-eight secures the bandage better than a simple spiral.

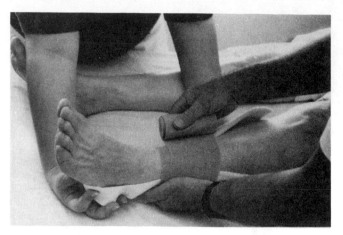

Figure 36–33

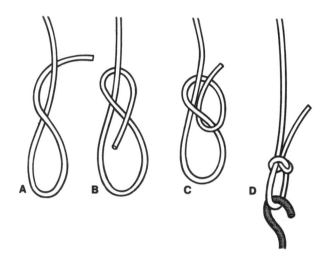

Figure 36–34
Tying a slip knot: **A**, make a figure eight; **B**, bring the free end of the rope through the lower loop; **C**, bring the free end of the rope under and through the upper loop; **D**, tighten the knot by pulling on the free end.

6. Secure the elastic bandage with adhesive tape.

7. Attach the spreader bar or footplate to the traction straps below the foot.

8. Tie the rope to whatever footpiece or spreader is being used. Use a slip knot which can be untied easily and rapidly. Figure 36–34 shows how to tie a slip knot.

9. Thread the rope through a pulley over the foot of the bed.

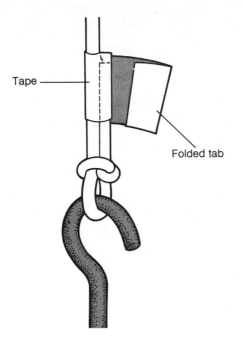

Tape

Folded tab

Figure 36–35

10. Using a slip knot, attach the end of the rope to a weight carrier.

11. Fasten the short ends of the ropes with tape to prevent them from slipping. When taping the ends of the ropes, make a folded tab at the end of the tape to facilitate its removal. See Figure 36–35.

12. Determine the amount of weight to be used and slowly place the weights on the carrier (see Figure 36–26).

    Rationale Sudden weight can jar the extremity and cause pain.

13. Assess neurovascular signs every 2–4 hours.

14. Remove and reapply the skin traction every 8 hours or more frequently as required to assess and maintain skin integrity.

PROCEDURE 36–18 **Assisting a Client in Traction**

After the application of traction, it is important for the nurse to assess the client's health as well as provide support. If the person has had skeletal traction applied in the operating room, postoperative care is usually needed as well.

EQUIPMENT

- Protective skin devices, eg, heel protectors.
- Trapeze if needed.
- Rubbing alcohol.
- Supplies for pin care in skeletal traction, eg, alcohol to clean the pin site or antiseptic recommended at the agency. Sterile technique is required.

INTERVENTION

1. Determine the degree of movement permitted and any special precautions, eg, bed positions permitted.

2. Inspect the traction apparatus regularly, ie, whenever you are at the bedside or at prescribed intervals, such as every 2 hours.
   Rationale Any articles that impinge on the traction can negate its effectiveness.

3. Provide protective devices and measures to safeguard the skin. For example, place heel protectors or sheepskins under the heels, sacrum, shoulders, and other pressure areas. Massage the skin with rubbing alcohol or lotion every 4 hours and, if redness and signs of pressure appear, every 2 hours.
   Rationale Alcohol tends to toughen the skin and leave it less vulnerable to breakdown. Since alcohol, however, is drying to the skin, lotion may be preferred for those who have dry skin (eg, elderly people).

4. Maintain the client in the supine position unless there are other orders.
   Rationale Changing position can change the body alignment and the amount of force supplied by the traction.

5. Maintain body alignment when turning the client. In some cases, the person can turn to a lateral position if body alignment is maintained by a

pillow placed between the legs. Refer to the client's record for information about permitted movement.

6. Provide a trapeze to assist the client to move and lift the body for back care if the person is unable to turn, eg, if the client has balanced suspension traction.

7. Do not remove skeletal and adhesive skin traction.
   Rationale A reduced fracture, for example, can become malpositioned if traction is removed; therefore, removal is a physician's responsibility.

8. Nonadhesive skin traction is intermittent and can be removed; check agency policy about any orders required. Remove the weights first; then unwrap the bandage and provide skin care. Rewrap the limb and slowly reattach the weights.

9. Provide pin site care. This varies with different authorities. Five principles recommended for such care are
   a. Carefully inspect the site
   b. Use sterile technique
   c. Remove crusts with a rolling technique
   d. Cover sites with a sterile barrier
   e. Determine frequency of care by the amount of drainage.
   Regular inspection of the pin site ensures early detection of minor infections, eg, serosanguineous drainage, crusting, swelling, and erythema. Sterile technique for cleaning helps protect the client from infection. Infection at the site can spread to the bone. Removing all crusted secretions permits the pin site to drain freely. Initial crusts around pins do not create a problem and can be left, but accumulated crusts around external fixator pins can cause secondary infection. These crusts can be removed by using ½ strength hydrogen peroxide twice daily. Using a gentle rolling technique reduces irritation to the tissue. The site is then covered with a sterile barrier, ie, sterile gauze or sterile ointment. One method is to soak 2 × 2 sterile gauze with povidone-iodine solution after the gauze has been applied around the pin. Procedures vary, so determine agency practices regarding pin site care.

10. Teach the client deep breathing and coughing to prevent hypostatic pneumonia.

11. Teach the client appropriate exercises to maintain and develop muscle tone, prevent muscle atrophy, and promote blood circulation. There are specific isometric exercises designed to strengthen the biceps and triceps muscles in preparation for using crutches. For example, raising the buttocks off the bed by pushing down with the arms develops the triceps, and pulling the body up with a trapeze develops the biceps. Isometric exercises to strengthen the quadriceps muscles include tightening the knees; by pushing the knees down without moving them the hamstring muscles are also strengthened. Tensing the buttocks and the inner thighs promotes stabilization of the hips; tensing the inner thighs also helps stabilize the knees. Circulation to the extremities is promoted by flexing and extending the feet as well as by the isometric exercises.

12. Document all assessments and nursing interventions.

PROCEDURE 36–19 **Turning a Client on a Stryker Wedge Frame**

Clients on turning frames are generally turned every 2 hours, but the frequency of turning depends on the person's health status, care requirements, and tolerance. The schedule for turning needs to be established with the client and recorded on the nursing care plan. The usual plan schedules turns so that the client can sleep on the posterior frame and have meals on the anterior one.

The procedure for turning a client on a standard Stryker frame is similar to that for the Stryker wedge frame discussed here, except that only *one* nurse is required for the Stryker wedge frame (see Figure 36–36). *Two* nurses are essential to turn the client on standard frames; one nurse stands at the foot, the other at the head, and on a signal the client is turned in unison. A third person may be required to ensure security of tubes and drains during turning.

EQUIPMENT

- The anterior or posterior frame, depending on the turn. These are usually kept at the bedside.
- Clean linen for the frame, as required. Special sheets with ties are available.
- Positioning devices, eg, pillow supports, footboards.
- Protective devices for the skin, eg, sheepskin.
- Incontinence pads, if required.
- Restraining straps.

INTERVENTION

1. Obtain baseline assessment data.

2. Even though the Stryker wedge frame can be operated by one nurse, it is a policy in many agencies that there should always be two nurses present when turning any bed frame.

3. Before turning the client, ensure that all nursing care requirements are completed. For example, if the client is on the posterior frame, the nurse can bathe all but the back and place a clean gown on the person.

4. Explain to the client the direction in which the turn will take place, eg, to the client's right or left.

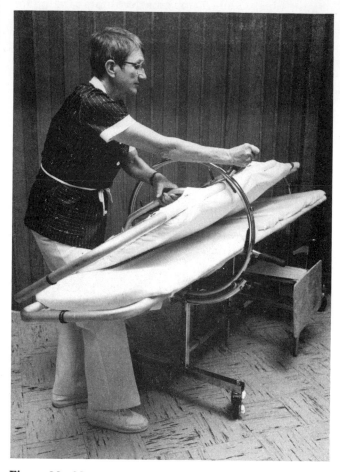

Figure 36–36
A Stryker wedge frame. Note the wedge shape formed by the anterior and posterior frames.

5. If the client has suction or drainage tubes, place this equipment carefully at the head of the bed before the turn. Be sure that the tubing is long enough to accommodate the turn. Place urinary drainage bags on the mattress beside the client; they must not pass above the client during the turn.

Turning from Supine to Prone Position

6. Ensure that the wheels of the frame are locked.
   Rationale The wheels are locked to prevent the frame from moving during the turn.

7. Remove the armboards and bed linen or bath blanket. Make sure the client's arms are not extended beyond the turning radius. If the client

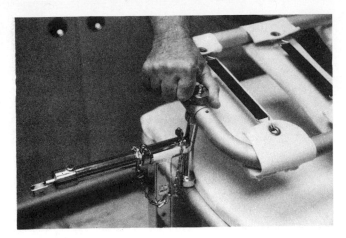

Figure 36–37

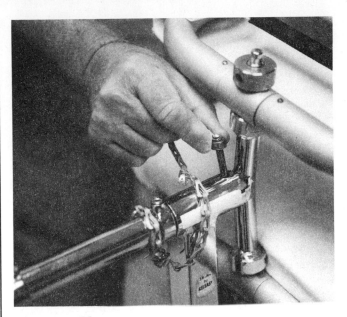

Figure 36–38

is unconscious do not remove the armboards until the arms are secured with straps.

8. Place a pillow lengthwise over the lower legs.
Rationale The pillow provides security during the turn and maintains the alignment of the feet and legs.

9. Ensure that the anterior frame has clean linen on it.

10. Place the anterior frame over the client, and tighten the knurled nut at the head of the frame. See Figure 36–37. The anterior frame will be angled with the posterior frame to form a wedge. If a standard Stryker frame is used, rather than the wedge frame, knurled nuts are fastened at *both* the head and the foot of the frame, and the frames are not angled.
Rationale Tightening the knurled nut(s) will keep the frame securely in place during the turn.

11. Ensure that the forehead and chin bands are placed appropriately, ie, that they do not obstruct the nose, mouth, and eyes. A pillow may be placed beside the head to prevent lateral movement during the turn.

12. Close the turning ring over the anterior frame, making sure that it is locked securely and that the frame fits snugly over the client. The nuts on the anterior turning ring can be adjusted to tighten the frame against the client. Directions for doing this are written on the frame.

13. Place the two restraining straps around both the frame and the client's legs and chest. Buckle the straps at the side of the client. If the standard Stryker frame is used, a third restraining strap is placed over the hips (on the wedge frame, the turning ring is positioned over the hips).

Rationale The straps prevent the client from slipping, especially the arms, if the client is unable to use them. Placing the strap buckle at the side makes it easier to open after the turn.

14. To turn the client:
   a. Ask the client to wrap both arms around the anterior frame, if able. Otherwise, make sure that the arms are restrained.
   Rationale This provides greater security when turning.
   b. Pull out the positive lock pin at the head of the frame. See Figure 36–38.
   Rationale The frame can pivot when this pin is out.
   c. Pull out the red turning lock knob on the turning ring. See Figure 36–39.
   Rationale This allows the frame to turn.
   d. Grasp the handle on the turning ring, and inform the client that you will turn on the count of 3. When two nurses are present the nurse at the head of the standard bed usually gives the directions for turning.
   e. Count to 3 and turn the frame toward you and toward the narrower side of the wedge, using a smooth, gradual motion.
   Rationale People feel more secure when turned toward the nurse.

15. Replace the positive lock pin.
Rationale The pin stabilizes the frame and prevents it from pivoting.

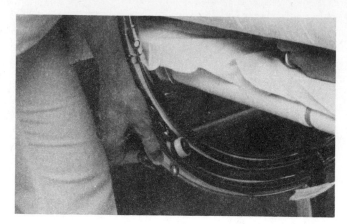

Figure 36–39

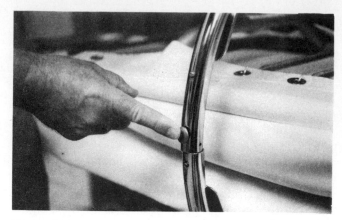

Figure 36–40

16. Push in the circular silver lock knob. See Figure 36–40. This opens the turning ring.

17. Release the knurled nut and remove the posterior frame.

18. Provide necessary care, and position the client.

Turning from Prone to Supine Position

19. Follow steps 1–7.

20. Place incontinence pads or sheepskins over the client's sacrum, if necessary, and put a small pillow under the lumbar curvature, if required.

21. Place the posterior frame over the person, and fasten it securely by tightening the knurled nut at the head of the frame.

22. Follow steps 12–17, and make the adjustments necessary for the person moving from the prone to the supine position.

For Either Position

23. Provide skin care to pressure areas as required.

24. Position the client in correct body alignment. Determine the physician's and nursing orders about the positioning supports that are recommended and permitted. Footboards are generally attached to prevent foot drop when the client is in the supine position. When the client is prone, the feet should hang over the end of the canvas in a flexed position. To prevent external rotation of the hips, a sandbag or trochanter roll may be placed against the hips.

25. Attach the armboards, and position the client's arms appropriately to prevent adduction contractures of the shoulders and flexion contractures of the elbows. The armboards should be slightly below the level of the frame when the client is in the prone position and level with the frame when the client is in the supine position.

26. Cover the client appropriately for warmth.

27. Place restraining straps around the client as a protective measure if required. Generally, one restraining strap is placed around the hips for clients receiving narcotics or sedatives and for all people at bedtime.

28. Instruct the client about foot or leg exercises, eg, dorsiflexion and plantar flexion, inversion and eversion of the foot, if health indicates.

29. Put clean linen and a pillow on the frame that was removed, in readiness for the next turn.

30. Document relevant assessments and interventions on the appropriate records.

PROCEDURE 36–20 **Turning a Client on a CircOlectric Bed**

A CircOlectric bed can turn 210°, thus permitting a client to assume a variety of positions. As Figure 36–41 shows, it consists of the following:

- An electrically operated circular framework and motor, which can be operated manually in case of a power failure.

- A posterior (basic) frame, for lying in the supine position, with a foam mattress, a mattress cover, and a headboard. A circular section of the mattress and a metal plate under the perineal area can be removed to insert a bedpan. The bedpan is held in place by special fasteners.

- An anterior frame, for lying in the prone position, with a foam mattress and cover.

- Special sheets that fasten to the mattresses with elastic bands.

- A footboard that attaches to the frame.

- A control switch to adjust the bed and a hand crank if it needs to be operated manually. The control switch has two labels, "Face" and "Back." The face switch turns the bed slowly to the prone position while the back switch turns it to supine position.

- Adjustable side rails.

- Forehead and chin supports for the anterior frame.

- Accessory equipment includes traction bars, an IV pole, exercise apparatus, and canvas arm slings to support the arms.

Before placing a client on a bed, the bed must be prepared. Cover the mattress sections with the special sheets, and lock the wheels to prevent the bed from rolling. Test the bed to make sure it is in good working order before the client is placed on it. It is important to explain to the client and support persons how the bed works. If possible, give a demonstration of the bed before the client is moved. Then lift the person onto the posterior frame. A person may be required to hold the head of a client who has had a neck injury and cannot control head movements. Center the person on the frame so that the buttocks are over the bedpan opening. Adjust the footboard to the client's height, and place pillows and rolls as needed to support the body in correct alignment.

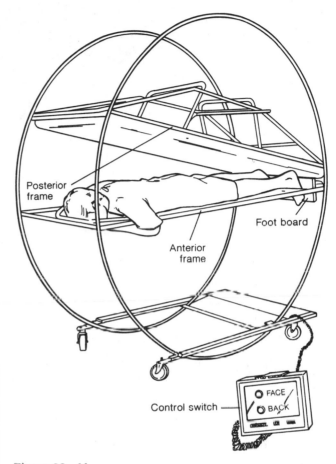

Figure 36–41
Some of the functional parts of a CircOlectric bed.

EQUIPMENT

- Restraining straps for the client in a prone position (side rails cannot be used)

- Canvas slings and/or safety belt to protect the client's arms if they cannot be held around the frame

- Skin care materials, including padding for bony prominences, if needed

- Positioning devices, eg, pillows, folded bath blankets, towels

INTERVENTION

1. Obtain baseline assessment data.

2. Lock the wheels of the bed.

   Rationale Locking the wheels will prevent the bed from moving during turning.

3. Describe the procedure and the sensations the client may experience. People often need considerable reassurance the first few times they are turned, because they experience vertigo (dizziness) from the turning. They also feel helpless and sometimes imagine that they will fall. It is important to discuss these sensations and reassure them that the turning is carefully controlled and can be stopped at any time.

4. Free any tubing, and arrange tubing and containers appropriately prior to the turn.

   Rationale Tubing can become tangled during the turn if it is not arranged beforehand.

5. Maintain eye contact with the client during any turn.

   Rationale Maintaining eye contact is reassuring to the client and allows the nurse to become immediately aware of any problem.

6. Do not stop a turn until the client reaches the intended position unless absolutely necessary.

   Rationale Stopping and starting a turn can increase a client's nausea and vertigo.

7. Maintain traction (eg, skull tongs) during the turn.

   Rationale Lack of traction can result in nonalignment of the vertebral column.

Turning from Supine to Upright or Prone Position

8. Measure the distance from the client's shoulders to ankles, and adjust the canvas of the anterior frame to fit the body.

   Rationale The anterior frame should support the body from the shoulders to the ankles.

9. Remove the restraining strap and top covers from the client.

10. Place a pillow or folded bath blanket lengthwise over the lower legs.

    Rationale This padding maintains their alignment and prevents movement during the turn.

11. Remove the pillow under the head.

12. Place the anterior frame over the client and fasten the bolts at both ends. See Figure 36–42.

13. Adjust the head support, and pad it if necessary.

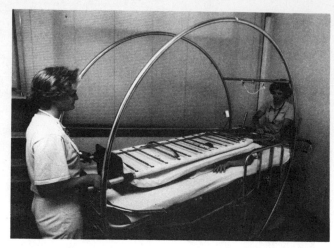

Figure 36–42
A CircOlectric bed with the anterior frame in place.

14. Make sure the client's feet are placed where they will not be injured by the footboard.

15. Assist the client to place both arms around the anterior frame. If the client cannot grasp the frame, place the arms alongside the body and secure them with a restraining strap, or place the arms in the canvas slings. See Figure 36–43.

16. Inform the client, then turn on the control marked "Face." The bed will move slowly, turning the client toward a prone position. (For an upright position, stop the bed when the client is vertical. The upright position is first established with the anterior frame in place. When the person tolerates standing between the frames for 5–10 minutes, the client then progresses to standing with only restraining straps at the waist and the knee.)

17. Release the switch when the client is in position, ie, horizontal.

18. Release the locks on the posterior frame, and push the frame upward until it locks in its gatched (raised) position.

19. Adjust the client's body to ensure correct alignment.

20. Place a restraining strap on the client to prevent a fall.

    Rationale The side rails cannot be used in the prone position, but a restraining strap offers a sense of security and will prevent the client from falling off the bed.

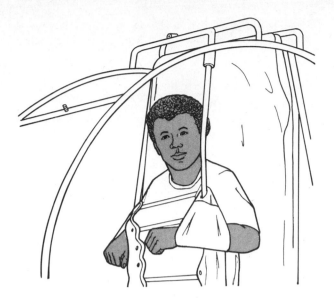

Figure 36–43

Turning from Prone to Supine Position

21. Remove the restraining strap and the bedclothes from the client.

22. Make sure that the footboard is placed against the feet.

    Rationale The footboard helps to stabilize the client during the turn.

23. Disengage the posterior frame from its raised position by releasing the lock and pushing the frame upward.

24. Lower the frame so that it fits over the client, then fasten the bolts at both ends.

25. Secure the client's arms as in step 15.

26. Inform the client, then turn on the control marked "Back." The bed will move slowly to turn the client toward a supine position.

27. Release the switch when the bed is horizontal or in the desired position.

28. Release the locks on the anterior frame, and remove the frame.

29. Remove the pillow or bath blanket over the legs.

30. Adjust the body for correct alignment. Provide supports, eg, a head pillow, as required.

31. Adjust the side rails, if necessary.

For All Turns

32. Provide skin care to bony prominences before and after the turn.

    Rationale Skin care before a turn will treat the pressure areas onto which the client will be moved; after a turn it will treat pressure areas the client has been lying on.

33. Adjust the bedclothes.

34. Assess the client's response to the turn in terms of discomfort, vertigo, syncope, nausea, and pallor.

35. Document relevant assessments and interventions. In many agencies, turns are recorded in a summary statement at the end of a shift.

Sample Recording

Date	Time	Notes
11/6/89	1600	Alternated prone and supine positions. A 5 cm diameter area on sacrum remains reddened, no breaks in the skin. No discomfort with turns, but states still fearful. ————Metsa C. Iwasaki, RN

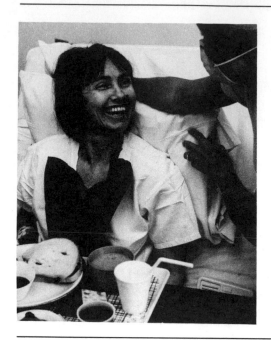

CHAPTER 39

NUTRITION

☐ The following procedures appear in *Introduction to Nursing:*

■ New procedures:

During illness or injury, the body often requires more nutrients than usual. Yet, because of illness or age, many clients are unable to feed themselves part or all of a meal. Thus, nurses need to become skillful in assisting clients to eat. Because patterns of eating vary considerably among people, the nurse needs to determine each person's food habits when planning nursing care. The nurse also needs to be able to assess the nutritional status of clients. To meet learning needs, nurses may teach new parents how to breast- or bottle-feed their infants.

PROCEDURE 39–2 **Assisting an Adult to Eat**

Some people who are ill require assistance eating. How much and what kind of assistance is needed depend on the physical and mental limitations of the person. Two groups of people frequently require help: the elderly, who are weakened and quickly fatigued when they are ill; and the handicapped (eg, blind people), those who must remain in a back-lying position, or those who do not have use of their hands. The client's nursing care plan will indicate that assistance is required with meals.

Because adults are normally able to eat independently, they may find assistance of any kind embarrassing and difficult to accept. Often clients become depressed because they require help and because they believe they are burdensome to busy nursing personnel. It is very important not to convey either verbally or nonverbally impatience or annoyance while assisting people to eat. Rather, appear unhurried and convey that you have ample time.

EQUIPMENT

- A meal tray with the correct food and fluids.

- An extra napkin or small towel to protect the client's clothes and the bedclothes.

- A straw, special drinking cup, or weighted glass if the client has difficulty taking fluids. See Figure 39–1.

INTERVENTION

1. Assess client for specific capabilities and to determine exact assistance required.

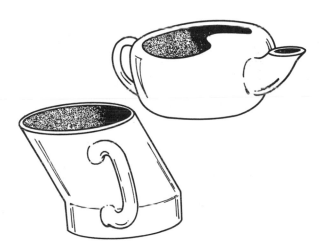

Figure 39–1
Two types of special drinking cups.

2. Assist the client to a sitting position, if possible, or to a lateral position if he or she is unable to sit.

   Rationale A person will swallow more easily in these positions than in a back-lying position.

3. If possible, assume a sitting position beside the client.

   Rationale The nurse's sitting conveys a more relaxed presence, which is more conducive to eating.

4. Assist the client to identify the food on the tray, if needed. For a blind person, identify the placement of the food as you would describe the time on a clock. See Figure 39–2.

5. Ask the order in which the client desires to eat the food.

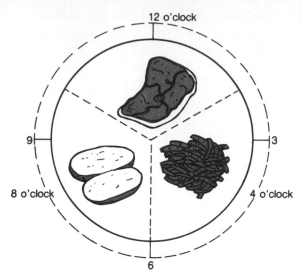

Figure 39-2

6. Use normal utensils whenever possible.

   Rationale Using ordinary utensils enhances self-esteem.

7. Encourage the person to eat independently, assisting where needed. Do not take over the feeding process.

   Rationale Participation enhances feelings of independence.

8. Warn the client if the food is hot or cold.

9. If the client cannot see, tell which food you are giving.

10. Allow ample time for the client to chew and swallow the food before offering more.

11. Provide fluids as requested, or, if the client is unable to talk, offer fluids after every three or four mouthfuls of solid food.

12. Use a straw or special drinking cup for fluids that would spill from normal containers.

13. Make the time a pleasant one, choosing topics of conversation that are of interest to the client, if the person wants to talk.

14. Demonstrate any new skills required and encourage practice. For example, the client may need to learn to cut food with one hand or to use only the nondominant hand.

15. After the meal, assist the client to clean the mouth and hands.

16. Document the amount of fluids taken, if fluid intake and output are monitored.

17. Document assessments (eg, the exact amounts of food consumed if a calorie count is needed) or if the client is anorexic or nauseated.

≋ Considerations for the Elderly

An overwhelming number of elderly people have one or more chronic illnesses or problems such as digestive upsets, lack of teeth or poorly fitting dentures, malabsorptive problems, osteoporosis, atherosclerosis, obesity, and alcohol addiction. It is a challenge to the nurse to identify problems that affect the client's nutrition status and in addition establish an appropriate nutrition program for the client.

Caloric intake should be reduced for all people as they become older because of the decrease in physical activity and basal metabolism of older adults. At the same time some elderly people require a higher carbohydrate intake. The specific nutrition requirements for older adults is a highly individualized matter. Most will require diets high in fiber and low in saturated fats and cholesterol. In addition, some will require meals that are bland, low in salt, or specialized (eg, diabetic diets). Some elderly people have decreased senses of smell and taste which contribute to a lack of appetite. When offering nutrition guidance, the nurse must also consider socioeconomic and cultural factors.

Because food and the eating experience have multiple facets (eg, physical survival, social involvement, and psychologic function), nutrition programs for the aged need to include more than a balance of nourishing foods. They also need to include some opportunity for meaningful social involvement and some opportunity for the person to choose and prepare foods. Nurses also need to be aware that eating habits that appear unhealthful to the nurse may be serving an important psychologic function for the older person. For instance, an older woman may not eat cheese because she believes it is the cause of her constipation.

PROCEDURE 39–3	**Administering a Gastrostomy or Jejunostomy Feeding**

Gastrostomy and jejunostomy feedings are used as alternatives to intravenous infusions and nasogastric feedings. They allow the client greater mobility and enable self-feedings. Jejunal feedings contain nutrients that can be absorbed in the small intestine without gastric and duodenal digestive processes. All feedings generally contain 1 kcal/mL of solution with protein, fat, carbohydrate, minerals, and vitamins in specified proportions. The solution is warmed in a basin of warm water or left to stand for a while until it reaches room temperature. Feedings are generally administered at room temperature unless the order specifies otherwise.

EQUIPMENT

- The correct amount of feeding solution. Amounts are gradually increased from 200–800 mL. Check the expiration date on a commercially prepared formula or the preparation date and time if the solution has been prepared in the agency. Discard a solution that has passed the expiration date or an agency formula that is more than 24 hours old.
- A large bulb syringe.
- A graduated container to hold the feeding.
- A graduated container with 60 mL of water to flush the tubing.

For a tube sutured in place:

- Some 4 × 4 gauze squares to cover the end of the tube.
- An elastic band.

For tube insertion:

- Water-soluble lubricant to lubricate the tube.
- Clean disposable gloves.
- A #18 Fr. whistle-tip catheter or other feeding tube.
- A tubing clamp.
- A moistureproof bag.

For a prosthesis:

- Water-soluble lubricant.
- A #18 Fr. whistle-tip catheter or other feeding tube.

For cleaning the peristomal skin and dressing the stoma:

- Mild soap and water.
- Petrolatum, zinc oxide ointment, or other skin protectant.
- Precut 4 × 4 gauze squares.
- Uncut 4 × 4 gauze squares.
- Abdominal pads.
- An abdominal binder or Montgomery straps.

INTERVENTION

1. Obtain baseline assessment data.

2. Provide privacy for this procedure. Gastrostomy and jejunal feedings involve exposing the abdomen, which is embarrassing to many people, and this method of feeding may in itself be embarrassing.

3. Assist the client to a Fowler's position in bed, a sitting position on a chair, or, if sitting is contraindicated, a slightly elevated right lateral position.
   Rationale These positions promote digestion and prevent esophageal reflux of a gastric feeding.

4. If a tube is already in place:
   a. Remove the gauze from the end of the tube.
   b. Attach the bulb syringe to the tube before unclamping the tube.
      Rationale A clamped tube prevents excess air from distending the stomach or duodenum and causing discomfort.
   c. Remove the clamp from the tube.
   d. Pour 15–30 mL of water into the syringe, remove the tube clamp, and allow the water to flow into the tube.
      Rationale This determines the patency of the tube. If water flows freely, the tube is patent; if it does not, notify the nurse in charge and/or physician.

5. If a tube is not in place, and one needs to be inserted:
   a. Lubricate the insertion end of the tube.

    b. Wearing gloves, remove the ostomy dressing. Discard the dressing and gloves in the moistureproof bag.

    c. Insert the tube into the ostomy opening 10–15 cm (4–6 in.).

6. If a prosthesis is in place:

    a. Remove the screw cap on the prosthesis.

    b. Lubricate and insert the feeding tube into the ostomy opening 10–15 cm (4–6 in.).

7. Aspirate and measure the stomach or jejunal contents as follows:

    a. Attach the bulb to the syringe and compress the bulb.

    Rationale Compressing the bulb before the syringe is attached to the feeding tube prevents the instillation of air into the stomach.

    b. Attach the syringe to the end of the feeding tube and withdraw the stomach or jejunal contents.

    c. Measure the amount of aspirated contents in a graduated pitcher.

    Rationale To evaluate absorption of the previous feeding, the aspirated amount is compared with the amount instilled. If the amount is significant (eg, more than half of the last feeding) the amount or frequency of the feeding may be changed.

    d. If 50 mL or more of undigested formula is withdrawn, check with the nurse in charge before proceeding.

    Rationale At some agencies a feeding is withheld if 50 mL or more of formula remains in the stomach to prevent nausea, vomiting, aspiration, and gastric dilatation.

    e. Reinstill the gastric or jejunal contents if this is the agency or the physician's practice. Remove the bulb and pour the contents via the syringe into the tube.

    Rationale The removed formula is reinstilled to prevent electrolyte imbalance.

8. To administer the feeding solution:

    a. Hold the syringe 7–15 cm (3–6 in.) above the ostomy opening.

    b. Slowly pour the solution into the syringe, and allow it to flow through the tube by gravity.

    c. Just before all the formula has run through and the syringe is empty, add 30 mL of water.

    Rationale Water rinses the tube and preserves its patency.

    d. If the tube is sutured in place, hold it upright, remove the syringe, and then clamp the tube to prevent leakage. Cover the end of the tube with a 4 × 4 gauze, and secure the gauze with a rubber band.

    e. If the tube was inserted for the feeding, remove it, and either apply the screw cap to a prosthesis or apply a dressing over the ostomy.

9. After the feeding, have the client remain in the sitting position or a slightly elevated right lateral position for at least 30 minutes.

    Rationale This prevents leakage and enhances the normal digestive process.

10. Assess status of peristomal skin. Gastric or jejunal drainage contains digestive enzymes that can irritate the skin. Any redness and broken skin areas need to be documented.

11. Check orders about cleaning the peristomal skin, applying a skin protectant, and applying appropriate dressings. Generally, the peristomal skin is washed with mild soap and water at least once daily. Petrolatum, zinc oxide ointment, or other skin protectant may be applied around the stoma, and precut 4 × 4 gauze squares may be placed around the tube. The precut squares are then covered with regular 4 × 4 gauze squares, and the tube is coiled over them. The coiled tube is covered with abdominal pads and secured with either an abdominal binder or Montgomery straps.

12. Document all assessments and interventions.

13. When appropriate, instruct the client about self-care of the stoma and tube, and how to administer a feeding.

PROCEDURE 39–4 **Establishing and Monitoring TPN Therapy**

Meticulous client monitoring is necessary during total parenteral nutrition (TPN) to prevent complications and to detect the effect on the client. Significant changes occur in the client's fluid, electrolyte, glucose, amino acid, vitamin, and mineral levels.

Many of the sepsis problems associated with conventional IV therapy are also associated with TPN. Moreover, the problems are magnified because: (a) clients receiving TPN therapy are often critically ill, may be malnourished, and are sometimes immunosuppressed; (b) TPN catheters are left in place for long periods of time; (c) the intralipids used in TPN therapy support the growth of a wide variety of microorganisms; and (d) the therapy uses the central venous system because of the osmolarity of the fluid. Infection control is therefore of utmost importance during TPN therapy.

EQUIPMENT

- The TPN (IVH) solution ordered

INTERVENTION

1. Obtain baseline assessment data.

Establishing the Infusion

2. Remove the ordered TPN solution from the refrigerator 1 hour before use, and check each ingredient and the proposed rate against the order on the chart.
   Rationale Infusion of a cold solution can cause pain, hypothermia, and venous spasm and constriction.

3. Inspect the solution for cloudiness or presence of particles, and ensure that the container is free from cracks.

4. After correct placement of the TPN catheter is confirmed by x-ray examination, change the solution container from the normal saline or dextrose solution to the TPN solution ordered.

Monitoring the Infusion

5. Inspect the catheter tubing for leaks and obstructions.

6. Inspect the catheter insertion site for signs of infiltration, eg, swelling.
   Rationale Infiltration of TPN solution can cause necrosis of tissues and sloughing of the dermis and epidermis.

7. Observe the client for signs of thrombosis or thrombophlebitis at the catheter insertion site (eg, edema or redness) and along the course of the vein (eg, pain or swelling of the arm, neck, or face). Purulent thrombophlebitis may result in a purulent discharge, which appears at the insertion site with slight pressure. If you observe such signs, notify the physician, who may order removal of the catheter and initiation of a heparin infusion at a peripheral vein site.

8. Monitor the vital signs every 4 hours. If fever or abnormal vital signs occur, notify the physician.
   Rationale An elevated temperature is one of the earliest indications of catheter-related sepsis.

9. Inspect the dressing every 4 hours for intactness, cleanliness, and presence of bleeding. Change the dressing at least every 48 hours, or more often if it is moist or loose, in accordance with agency policy. See Procedure 39–6.

10. Change the IV tubing every 24 hours or in accordance with agency policy. See Procedure 39–5.

11. Always practice strict surgical aseptic technique when changing solutions, tubing, filters, and dressings.

12. Always check agency policies and procedures before you (a) take central venous pressure (CVP) measurements, (b) take blood samples, (c) piggyback other solutions, or (d) inject medications.

13. Before administering any TPN solution, check its expiration date. Most solutions must be used within 24 hours of preparation, unless they are refrigerated.

14. Carefully monitor the infusion flow rate and the laboratory test results to detect complications such as hyperglycemia or electrolyte imbalance. Use of an infusion pump keeps the infusion rate regular.

15. Collect double-voided urine specimens at least every 6 hours or in accordance with agency policy, and test the urine for specific gravity and

glucose and acetone levels. If the specific gravity is abnormal, notify the physician, who may alter the constituents of the TPN solution. Also notify the physician if the glucose level is elevated to 2% (++). Supplementary insulin may be ordered and given subcutaneously or added directly to the TPN solution by pharmacy personnel.

Rationale Glucosuria is often the first sign of catheter-related sepsis.

16. Document the daily fluid intake and output and calorie intake as baseline data. Precise replacement for fluid and electrolyte deficits can then be more readily determined.

17. Weigh the client daily, at the same time and in the same garments. A gain of more than 0.5 kg (1.1 lb) per day indicates fluid excess and should be reported. Measure arm circumference and triceps skin fold thickness to assess the physical changes.

18. Monitor the results of laboratory tests (eg, serum electrolytes, blood glucose, and blood urea nitrogen) and report abnormal findings to the physician.

PROCEDURE 39–5 **Changing TPN Tubing**

The CDC recommends that TPN tubing be changed at least once every 24–48 hours. Some experts advise that it be changed every 24 hours. This procedure is best carried out when the TPN solution container is being changed. Strict surgical aseptic technique must be practiced.

EQUIPMENT

- Sterile gloves
- Mask
- Sterile 2 × 2 gauze squares to place under the tubing–catheter connection site and to clean the junction of the catheter and tubing, if agency practice indicates
- A new solution container and administration set (tubing)
- Tape to secure the tubing to the catheter
- Antiseptic to clean the catheter and tubing junction as agency practice indicates

INTERVENTION

1. Obtain baseline assessment data.
2. Assist the client to the supine position.
   Rationale This lowers the negative pressure in the vena cava, thus decreasing the risk of air embolism when the catheter is opened.
3. Prepare the solution container, attach the new IV tubing, and prime the tubing as you would for a conventional IV.
4. Wash hands as required before handling sterile supplies.
5. Remove the tape securing the tubing to the dressing and the catheter hub connection.

6. Open the package containing the sterile gauze squares.
7. Don sterile gloves.
8. Place the sterile gauze underneath the connection site of the catheter and tubing. Clean the junction of the catheter and tubing.
   Rationale This prevents the transfer of microorganisms from the client's skin to the open TPN catheter tip when it is detached; it also decreases the number of microorganisms at the catheter-tubing junction.
9. Ask the client to perform Valsalva's maneuver and to turn the head away while detaching the IV tubing by rotating it out of the hub.
   Rationale Performance of Valsalva's maneuver reduces the risk of air embolism and turning the head to the side reduces the chances of contaminating the equipment.
10. Quickly attach the new primed IV tubing to the TPN catheter, ensuring a tight seal.
    Rationale The tubing must be attached quickly while the client is performing the Valsalva maneuver.
11. Open the clamp on the new tubing, and adjust the flow to the rate ordered.
12. Secure the tubing to the catheter with tape if a Leur-Lok connection is not present.
    Rationale This prevents accidental separation of the tubes and contamination of the TPN system.
13. Loop and tape the tubing over the dressing.
    Rationale This prevents tension on the catheter and inadvertent separation of tubing and catheter.
14. Mark the date and time of the tubing change on the new IV tubing or drip chamber.
15. Document the tubing change and all assessments.

PROCEDURE 39–6 **Changing a TPN Dressing**

Nurses need to change TPN dressings every 48–72 hours and more frequently if a dressing becomes wet or loose. The high glucose concentration of the TPN solution makes the hyperalimentation insertion site very vulnerable to infection. Meticulous asepsis and dressing changes are essential to prevent infection.

EQUIPMENT

A sterile dressing kit containing:

- Gloves (2 pairs).
- Some 4 × 4 gauze sponges for cleaning and dressing application.
- Tissue forceps (optional) for cleaning.
- Solution bowls for the cleaning solutions.
- Precut drain gauze (optional).
- A 2 × 2 gauze for the insertion site.
- Two face masks (one for the nurse and one for the client).
- Isopropyl alcohol.
- Antiseptic solutions. Usually 10% acetone and 1% iodine tincture or povidone-iodine solutions are used. If the client is allergic to iodine, substitute 70% alcohol. Swabs may be prepackaged in the sterile kit.
- Povidone-iodine ointment. If the client is allergic to iodine, substitute a combination of antimicrobial and antifungal agents.
- Tincture of benzoin. This may be available in a spray container.
- Sterile scissors to cut gauze for the drain site, if precut gauze is not available.
- Elastoplast tape or transparent occlusive dressing such as Op-Site, to cover the gauze dressings.
- Nonallergenic 2.5-cm (1-in.) tape to secure the Elastoplast.
- A waterproof bag for used dressings and supplies.

INTERVENTION

1. Determine whether the client is allergic to iodine or tape.

2. Assist the client to a supine or a semi-Fowler's position.

3. Don a mask and have the client don a mask (if tolerated or as agency policy indicates) and ask the client to turn the head away from the insertion site.

   Rationale This helps protect the TPN insertion site from the nurse's and client's nasal and oral microorganisms. Turning the client's head also makes the site more accessible.

4. Clean the client's overbed table with isopropyl alcohol, and allow it to air dry.

5. Wash hands as before handling sterile supplies and, if agency policy indicates, apply alcohol and allow the hands to air dry.

6. Open the sterile supplies on the clean overbed table, and fill the solution bowls with the required solutions, if indicated.

7. If iodine ointment is used, squeeze some of it onto a corner of a sterile gauze.

8. Remove the soiled dressing by pulling the tape slowly and gently from the skin.

   Rationale This prevents catheter displacement and skin irritation.

9. Inspect the skin for signs of irritation or infection. Inspect the catheter for signs of leakage or other problems. If infection is suspected, take a swab of the drainage for culture, label it, send it to the laboratory, and notify the physician.

10. Don sterile gloves.

11. Clean the catheter insertion site with sterile gauze sponges soaked in a solvent such as 10% acetone. Clean in a circular motion, moving from the insertion site outward to the edge of the adhesive border. Take care not to jostle or get acetone on the catheter. Take a new sponge for each wipe. Repeat until the sponge is unstained after use.

    Rationale Acetone defats the skin, destroys bacterial cell walls, and removes old adhesive tape, which would irritate the skin if left on. Cleaning from the insertion site outward and discarding sponges after each wipe avoids introducing contaminants from the uncleaned area to the site. Jostling the catheter can cause discomfort to the client and could dislodge the catheter. Acetone is kept off the catheter because it could corrode the catheter.

12. Using the method in step 11, clean the insertion site and catheter for 2 minutes with povidone-iodine solution or iodine tincture. Focus on the insertion site, and allow the iodine to air dry for at least 30 seconds. If using 70% alcohol as a substitute for iodine, clean the area for 5 minutes.

    Rationale The iodine solution is an antiseptic with antimicrobial properties that last a long time, even after drying.

13. Ensure that the connection of the catheter to the IV tubing is secure, if it is within the dressing site.

14. Remove your gloves, and put on the other sterile pair.

    Rationale The gloves used for cleaning are considered contaminated.

15. Continue to clean the skin with povidone-iodine solution for 3 minutes or with alcohol solution for 5 minutes. Follow agency practice about cleaning and drying times.

16. Apply the povidone-iodine ointment to the insertion site and to the catheter hub, taking care not to loosen the catheter-tubing connection.

17. If the catheter is taped in place, ensure that the tape is clean. If the tape is soiled, remove and replace it with sterile tape, using the crisscross (chevron) taping method. See Figure 39–3.

18. Apply the precut sterile drain gauze around the catheter. See Figure 39–4. (If precut gauze is not available, cut a 2 × 2 sterile gauze square, using the sterile scissors.) Apply sufficient sterile gauze dressings to cover the catheter and skin.

    Rationale This protects the catheter and skin surrounding the insertion site from airborne contaminants.

19. If using Elastoplast dressing, apply tincture of benzoin to the skin surrounding the dressing gauzes and allow it to air dry about 1 minute.

    Rationale This protects the skin when adhesive tape or Elastoplast is applied and promotes adhesion of the cover dressing. Appropriate drying time is essential or skin breakdown can occur when the dressing is removed.

20. Remove your gloves.

21. Ask the client to abduct the arm and turn the head away from the dressing site. Tape the dressing securely to the skin with Elastoplast or trans-

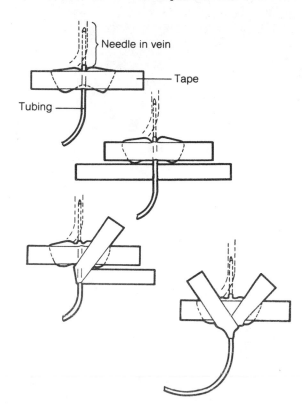

Figure 39–3

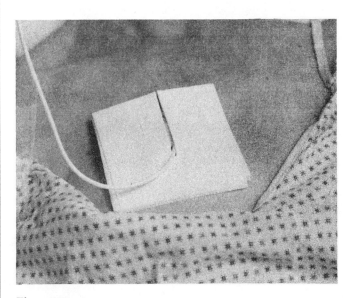

Figure 39–4

parent occlusive dressing. Make sure that the adhesive covering is occlusive, as is the dressing shown in Figure 39–5.

Rationale Arm abduction and head rotation ensure that the client's range of motion is not limited by the adhesive dressing and decrease the potential for skin abrasion caused by movement of the adhesive.

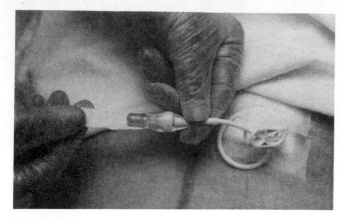

Figure 39-5

22. Loop and tape the IV tubing (not the filter) over the occlusive dressing.

    Rationale Looping prevents tension on the catheter and its inadvertent detachment if the tubing is pulled.

23. Label a strip of tape with the date, time, and the nurse's initials, and apply it to the dressing.

24. Document the dressing change and all assessments.

Variation: Changing a Dressing for a Surgically Inserted Central Venous Line

The distal end of a central venous catheter lies on the chest somewhere between the nipple and the sternum. The proximal tip lies in the right atrium of the heart. When the catheter is newly inserted, there are two sites that require dressing: the insertion site, where the catheter enters the vein, and the exit site, where the catheter leaves the chest. See Figure 39-6. Once the insertion site incision has healed, only the catheter exit site requires care.

The distal end of the catheter is threaded and has a male Luer-Lok cap. In some agencies the Luer-Lok cap is replaced with a special cap that has an injection port, which is also threaded. The cap is screwed

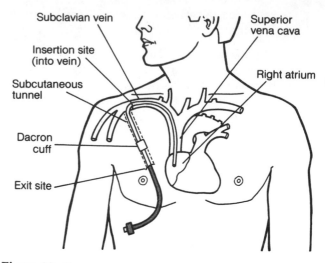

Figure 39-6
A Hickman catheter surgically inserted into the chest wall, entering the subclavian vein, and extending into the right atrium.

onto the catheter securely. Some authorities also recommend that the cap be taped to prevent it from dislodging or allowing an air embolus to enter. See Figure 39-5. Some authorities suggest that the catheter should have a smooth clamp in place continuously. The clamp must not have teeth, because they could damage the catheter. It is normally placed over tape on the line, as an added precaution against severing the catheter. The clamp is closed when the catheter is not being used.

The insertion site for the catheter is cleaned the way any surgical incision is cleaned until it is healed. The frequency of dressing changes varies among agencies; however, once every 24 or 48 hours is not unusual.

The exit site is also cleaned, and the dressing is changed until the site is completely healed. At that time practices vary at different agencies. At some, the healed exit site is left exposed to the air and cleaned with hydrogen peroxide only when it is soiled. Agencies also vary in choice of dressing materials.

PROCEDURE 39–7 **Obtaining a Capillary Blood Specimen and Measuring Blood Glucose**

A capillary blood specimen is often used to test the blood glucose level when frequent tests are required or when a venipuncture cannot be performed. This procedure is less painful than a venipuncture and easily performed. Hence, clients can perform this procedure upon themselves.

The development of home glucose test kits and reagent strips has simplified the testing of blood glucose. A number of manufacturers have developed blood glucose meters. Most permit measurements between 20 and 800 mg/100 mL of blood.

EQUIPMENT

- An antiseptic swab to cleanse the skin before the capillary puncture
- A cotton ball to wipe the glucose reagent strip
- A blood glucose meter (see Figure 39–7)
- A blood glucose reagent strip compatible with the monitor
- Paper towel
- Nonsterile disposable gloves for the nurse.

INTERVENTION

1. Obtain a reagent strip from the container.

2. Insert the strip into the meter according to the manufacturer's instructions and make any required adjustments.

    Rationale Some meters require calibration or the adjustment of the timer.

3. Remove the reagent strip from the meter and place it on a clean dry paper towel.

    Rationale Moisture can change the strip, thereby altering the test results.

4. Don gloves.

    Rationale It is likely that the nurse's hands will come in contact with the client's blood.

5. Choose a vascular puncture site, eg, the side of an adult's finger. Avoid sites beside bone.

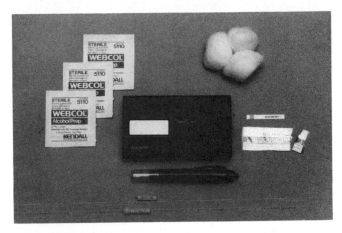

Figure 39–7
Equipment to measure capillary blood glucose. Clockwise around the glucose meter, from top left: antiseptic swabs, cotton balls, reagent strips, lancet and lancet holder.

6. Hold the finger in a dependent position while massaging toward the tip.

    Rationale These measures increase the blood supply to the area.

7. Clean the site with the antiseptic swab and permit it to dry.

8. Place the lancet or bloodletting device against the site and release the needle, thus permitting it to pierce the skin. Make sure the lancet is perpendicular to the site.

    Rationale The lancet is designed to pierce the skin at a specific depth when it is in a perpendicular position relative to the skin.

9. Wipe away the first drop of blood with a cotton ball.

    Rationale The first blood usually contains a greater proportion of serous fluid, which can alter test results.

10. Gently squeeze the site until a large drop of blood forms.

11. Transfer the drop of blood to the reagent strip, making sure it is on the test pad. The pad will absorb the blood and a chemical reaction will occur. Do not smear the blood as this will cause an inaccurate reading.

12. Press the timer on the glucose meter and monitor the time as indicated by the manufacturer, eg, 60 seconds. Lay the glucose strip on a paper towel.

    Rationale   The blood must remain in contact with the chemical for a prescribed time for accurate results.

13. Apply pressure to the skin puncture site by using a cotton ball.

    Rationale   Pressure will assist *hemostasis*.

14. When the timer displays the time indicated by the manufacturer, no blood should remain on the strip.

15. Place the strip into the meter while the timer continues.

16. At the designated time, eg, 120 seconds, activate the meter to display the glucose reading.

17. Turn off the meter and discard the test strip and cotton balls.

18. Remove and properly dispose of gloves.

19. Wash hands before documenting the results on the client's record.

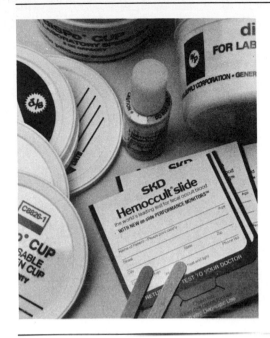

CHAPTER 40

FECAL ELIMINATION

☐ The following procedures appear in *Introduction to Nursing:*

Procedure 40–1
Obtaining and Testing a Specimen of Feces

Procedure 40–2
Administering an Enema

Procedure 40–3
Changing a Bowel Diversion Ostomy Appliance

■ New procedures:

Procedure 40–4
Removing a Fecal Impaction Digitally

Procedure 40–5
Irrigating a Colostomy

Elimination of the waste products of digestion is essential to health. Adequate elimination depends on the correct functioning of the small and large intestines, the nervous system, and the urinary system, as well as factors such as diet, exercise, fluid intake, and regularity.

Nurses are involved frequently in assisting clients with a variety of bowel and urinary problems brought about by illness, diagnostic tests, age, or faulty health habits. Common fecal elimination aids include the use of bedpans, the administration of enemas, and the insertion of rectal tubes or rectal suppositories. Less commonly, clients need help with irrigating bowel diversion ostomies.

PROCEDURE 40–4 **Removing a Fecal Impaction Digitally**

Fecal impaction is indicated by the passage of no stools, seepage of liquid feces, rectal pain, desire to defecate to no avail, and a general feeling of malaise. The nurse can confirm the presence of an impaction through digital examination of the rectum.

Although fecal impaction can generally be prevented, digital removal of impacted feces is sometimes necessary. When fecal impaction is suspected, the client is often given an oil retention enema, a cleansing enema 2–4 hours later, and daily additional cleansing enemas, suppositories, or stool softeners. If these measures fail, manual removal is necessary. This process involves breaking up the fecal mass digitally and removing it in portions. Because the bowel mucosa can be injured during this procedure, some agencies restrict and specify the personnel permitted to conduct digital disimpactions. Rectal stimulation is also contraindicated for some people since it may cause an excessive vagal response resulting in cardiac arrhythmia.

After a disimpaction, various interventions can be used to remove remaining feces, eg, a cleansing enema or the insertion of a suppository.

EQUIPMENT

- A moisture-resistant bedpad
- A bedpan and cover
- Toilet tissue
- Disposable gloves
- Lubricant

INTERVENTION

1. Obtain baseline assessment data.

2. Explain to the client what you plan to do and why. This procedure is distressing, tiring, and uncomfortable, so the person may desire the presence of another nurse or support person.

3. Assist the client to a right lateral or Sims' position with the back toward you.
   Rationale When lying on the right side, the sigmoid colon is uppermost; thus, gravity can aid removal of the feces.

4. Place the disposable bedpad under the client's hips, and arrange the top bedclothing so that it falls obliquely over the hips, exposing only the buttocks.

5. Place the bedpan and toilet tissue nearby on the bed or a bedside chair.

6. Put on the gloves.

7. Lubricate the gloved index finger.
   Rationale Lubricant reduces resistance by the anal sphincter as the finger is inserted.

8. Gently insert the index finger into the rectum, moving toward the umbilicus.

9. Gently massage around the stool.
   Rationale Gentle action prevents damage to the rectal mucosa. A circular motion around the rectum dislodges the stool and stimulates peristalsis, and relaxes the anal sphincter.

10. Work the finger into the hardened mass of stool to break it up. If you cannot break up the impaction with one finger, insert two fingers and try to break up the impaction scissor style.

11. Work the stool down to the anus, remove it in small pieces, and place them in the bedpan.

12. Carefully continue to remove as much fecal material as possible; at the same time assess the client for signs of pallor, feelings of faintness, shortness of breath, and perspiration. Terminate the procedure if these occur.

    Rationale Manual stimulation could result in excessive vagal nerve stimulation and subsequent cardiac arrhythmia.

13. Assist the client to a position on a clean bedpan, commode, or toilet.

    Rationale Digital stimulation of the rectum may induce the urge to defecate.

14. Document the removal of a fecal impaction and all assessments, eg, the appearance and amount of stool, and vital signs.

Sample Recording

Date	Time	Notes
9/28/89	1000	Rectal examination for fecal impaction. Moderate amount dark brown feces removed digitally. Vital signs stable. Unable to defecate following procedure. ————Bruce L. Ching, NS

15. If appropriate, teach the client measures to promote normal elimination. Alterations in diet and fluid intake and the use of stool softeners may be necessary.

PROCEDURE 40–5 **Irrigating a Colostomy**

A colostomy irrigation is similar to an enema. The purpose of irrigation is to distend the bowel sufficiently to stimulate peristalsis, which causes evacuation to occur.

The physician initially is responsible for determining whether a colostomy should be irrigated, what solution should be used, and the type and amount of irrigation to be given. The last may be preestablished by agency policy, however.

Routine daily irrigations done to control the time of elimination ultimately become the client's decision. Some people prefer to control the time of elimination by rigid dietary regulation and not be bothered with irrigations, which can take up to 1 hour to complete. When regulation by irrigation is chosen, it should be done at the same time each day. Control by irrigations also necessitates some control of the diet. For example, laxative foods that might cause an unexpected evacuation need to be avoided.

In most clients, a relatively small amount of fluid (300–500 mL) stimulates evacuation. In others, up to 1000 mL may be needed, since a colostomy has no sphincter and the fluid tends to return as it is instilled. This problem is reduced by the use of a cone on the irrigating catheter. The cone helps to hold the fluid within the bowel during the irrigation.

Irrigations are commonly used for end colostomies and descending colostomies; they are not advised for ascending colostomies or ileostomies, where the effluent is liquid in nature.

If the client has had a colostomy for a long time, the irrigation needs to be given at the time the client has established, or the pattern of regularity will be disrupted. For a newly established colostomy, select a time based on the client's previous bowel habits and one that will allow the client to participate in usual daily activities. Encourage the client to select the time and to maintain it.

EQUIPMENT

A variety of equipment is available for colostomy irrigation, but the basic components are

- A moisture-resistant bag for the soiled colostomy bag or dressings.

- A clean colostomy appliance or dressings.

- Irrigation equipment. See figures 40–1 and 40–2.

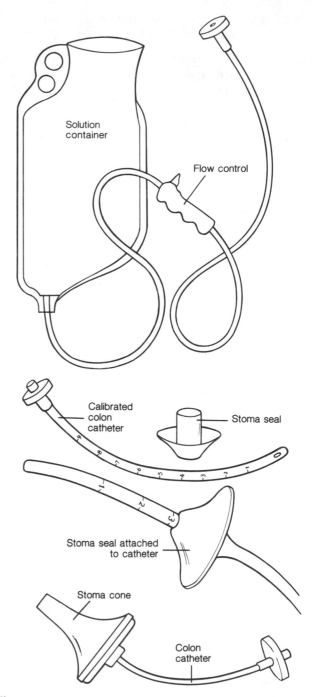

Figure 40–1
Colostomy irrigation equipment.

- A bag to hold the solution. For routine irrigations for regulation, the bag is usually filled with 500 mL of warm (body temperature) tap water, or other

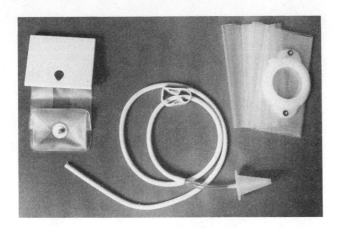

Figure 40–2
A commercially prepared colostomy irrigation set. The irrigation solution bag is on the left and the collecting bag (irrigation drainage sleeve) on the right; the stoma cone is fitted to the catheter.

solution as ordered. For a bowel preparation 1000 mL of solution is needed.

- Tubing attached to the bag.
- A tubing clamp or flow regulator.
- A #28 rubber colon catheter, which may be calibrated in either centimeters or inches, with a stoma or seal.
- A disposable stoma irrigation drainage sleeve with belt to direct the fecal contents into the toilet or bedpan.
- Lubricant.
- Clean rubber gloves to protect the nurse's hands from contamination, and one glove to dilate the stoma if ordered by the physician.
- A bath blanket to cover the client as required.
- An IV pole as required to suspend the irrigation bag.
- A disposable bedpad, bedpan, and cover, if the client is to remain in bed.

INTERVENTION

1. Determine the purpose of the irrigation and which stoma is to be irrigated. Usually, the proximal stoma is irrigated, to stimulate the bowel to evacuate. However, the physician may want the distal stoma irrigated as well in preparation for diagnostic procedures (eg, roentgenography). If there are two stomas, determine which is the distal and which is the proximal.

2. Before a colostomy irrigation:
   a. Assess the client's readiness to select and use the equipment. Because many types of irrigation sets are available, clients should begin with a "starter set" until they are familiar with the colostomy and the problems of irrigating it. Later, with the help of an enterostomal therapy nurse or a qualified person from a surgical supply house, the client can select the set that is most appropriate.
   b. Auscultate the abdomen for bowel sounds.
   c. Palpate the abdomen for distention.

3. Explain the procedure and its purpose. The total irrigation process usually takes about 1 hour.

4. Assist the client who is to remain in bed to a side-lying position, and place a disposable bedpad on the bed in front of the client. Place the bedpan on top of the disposable pad, beneath the stoma. Assist an ambulatory client to sit on the toilet or on a commode in the bathroom.

5. Ensure that the client's gown or pajamas are moved out of the way to prevent soiling, and drape the person appropriately with the bath blanket to prevent undue exposure. Throughout the technique provide explanations, and encourage the client to participate as much as the client desires.

6. Hang the solution bag on an IV pole so that the bottom of the container is at the level of the client's shoulder, or 30–45 cm (12–18 in.) above the stoma.
   Rationale This height provides a pressure gradient that allows fluid to flow into the colon. The rate of flow can be regulated by the tubing clamp.

7. Attach the colon catheter securely to the tubing.

8. Open the regulator clamp, and run fluid through the tubing to expel all air from it. Close the clamp until ready for the irrigation.
   Rationale Air distends the bowel and can cause cramps.

9. Don gloves.

10. Remove the soiled colostomy bag, and place it in the moisture-resistant bag.
    Rationale Placing the colostomy bag in such a container prevents the transmission of microorganisms and helps reduce odor.

11. Center the irrigation drainage sleeve over the stoma, and attach it snugly.
    Rationale This prevents seepage of the fluid onto the skin.

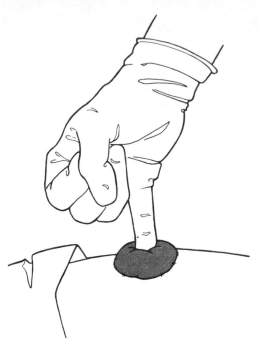

Figure 40–3

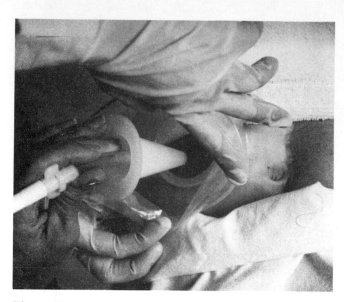

Figure 40–4
The client is participating in the irrigation by directing the cone.

12. Direct the lower open end of the drainage sleeve into the bedpan or between the client's legs into the toilet.

13. If ordered, dilate the stoma:
    a. Lubricate the tip of the little finger.
    b. Gently insert the finger into the stoma, using a massaging motion. See Figure 40–3.

    Rationale A massaging motion relaxes the intestinal muscles.

    c. Repeat steps a and b above, using progressively larger fingers until maximum dilation is achieved.

    Rationale Stoma dilation is performed to stretch and relax the stomal sphincter and to assess the direction of the proximal colon prior to an irrigation.

14. Lubricate the tip of the stoma cone or colon catheter.

    Rationale Lubricating the tip of the cone or catheter eases insertion and prevents injury to the stoma.

15. Using a rotating motion, insert the catheter or stoma cone through the opening in the top of the irrigation drainage sleeve and gently through the stoma. See Figure 40–4. Insert a catheter only 7 cm (3 in.); insert a stoma cone just until it fits snugly. Many practitioners prefer using a cone to avoid the risk of perforating the bowel. If you

have difficulty inserting the catheter or cone, do not apply force.

    Rationale A rotating motion on insertion helps to open the stoma. Forcing the cone or catheter may traumatize or perforate the bowel.

16. Open the tubing clamp, and allow the fluid to flow into the bowel. If cramping occurs, stop the flow until the cramps subside and then resume the flow.

    Rationale Fluid that is administered too quickly or is too cold may cause cramps. If the fluid flows out as fast as you put it in, press the stoma cone or seal more firmly against the stoma to occlude it. If a stoma cone or seal is not available, press around the stoma with your fingers to close the stoma against the catheter.

17. After all the fluid is instilled, remove the catheter or cone and allow the colon to empty. In some agencies the stoma cone is left in place for 10–15 minutes before it is removed. Although not always indicated, you may ask the client to gently massage the abdomen and sit quietly for 10–15 minutes until initial emptying has occurred.

    Rationale Massaging the abdomen encourages initial emptying.

18. Clean the base of the irrigation drainage sleeve, and seal the top and bottom with a drainage clamp, following the manufacturer's instructions.

19. Encourage an ambulatory client to move around for about 30 minutes.

    Rationale Complete emptying of the colon takes up to half an hour. Moving around facilitates peristalsis.

20. Empty the irrigator drainage sleeve, and remove it.

21. Clean the area around the stoma, and dry it thoroughly.

22. Put a colostomy appliance on the client as needed. (See Procedure 40–3 in *Introduction to Nursing*.)

23. Promptly report to the nurse in charge any problems, such as no fluid or stool returns, difficulties inserting the tube, peristomal skin redness or irritation, and stomal discoloration.

24. Document all assessments and interventions. Include the time of the irrigation, the type and amount of fluid instilled, the returns, and any problems experienced.

Sample Recording

Date	Time	Notes
12/5/89	0900	Colostomy irrigated with 750 mL warm tap water. Water and large amount soft brown stool expelled. Tube inserted without difficulty. Peristomal skin intact. Stoma is pink. Asked questions about irrigation, looked at stoma for first time. Observed stoma care and pouch application. ————————————Chung-Hao Jen, NS

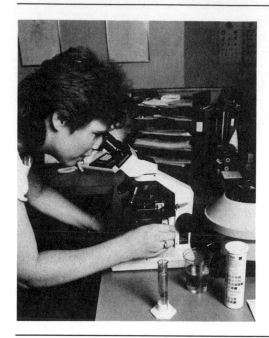

URINARY
ELIMINATION

The urinary system extends interiorly from the urinary meatus, along the urethra, into the urinary bladder, through the ureters, to the kidneys. This system normally does not contain microorganisms except at the urinary meatus; therefore, any techniques that introduce equipment into the urinary tract must be sterile. A urinary catheterization introduces a catheter into the urinary bladder, and a bladder irrigation also introduces fluid into the bladder. Peritoneal dialysis also requires surgical aseptic technique, although in this instance a catheter and solution (dialysate) are introduced into the peritoneal cavity to remove waste products normally excreted through the urinary system. Specimens of urine are collected routinely from hospital clients for a variety of tests.

PROCEDURE 41–9 Collecting a Timed Urine Specimen

Several urine tests require timed specimens. Urine specimens are collected at timed intervals, for short periods (1–2 hours) or long periods (12–24 hours). All timed urine specimens need to be refrigerated or kept on ice to prevent bacterial growth and decomposition of the urine components, which can affect the findings. For some timed specimens large collection containers are kept in a refrigerator, often in the laboratory—not at the bedside. Each voiding of urine is collected in a small clean container and then emptied immediately into the large refrigerated bottle. In most instances the entire amount of urine voided is collected.

For some tests a chemical urine preservative, eg, toluene or acetic acid, is added to the large collection container. Other tests require different preservatives, since certain additives invalidate the results for certain tests. It is wise to contact the laboratory prior to the specimen collection to confirm the additive for a test.

EQUIPMENT

- Appropriate specimen containers with or without preservative in accordance with the specific test. These are generally obtained from the laboratory and placed in the client's bathroom or in the utility room.

- Completed specimen identification labels. The labels need to indicate the date and time of each voiding in addition to the usual identification information. They may also be numbered sequentially, eg, 1st specimen, 2d specimen, 3d specimen.

- A completed laboratory requisition.

- A bedpan or urinal.

- An alert card indicating the specific times for urine collection. This is placed in the client's room, on or near the bed. It reminds all nursing staff that the test is in progress.

- An antiseptic.

INTERVENTION

1. Give explicit instructions about the purpose of the test and how the client can assist. Tell the client when the specimen collection will begin and end. For example, a 24-hour urine test commonly begins at 0700 hours and ends at the same hour the next day. Instructions should include the following facts:
   a. All urine must be saved and placed in the specimen containers once the test starts.
   b. The urine must be free of fecal contamination and toilet tissue.
   c. Each specimen must be given to the nursing staff immediately so that it can be placed in the appropriate specimen bottle.

2. Start the collection period by asking the client to void in the toilet or bedpan or urinal. Discard this urine (check agency procedure) and document the time the test starts with this discarded specimen. Collect all subsequent urine specimens, including the one at the end of the period.

3. Ask the client to ingest the required amount of liquid for certain tests.

4. Measure the urine, and inspect each specimen for color, odor, and characteristics.

5. Document the starting time of the test on the client's record.

6. Instruct the client to void all subsequent urine into the bedpan or urinal and to notify the nursing staff when each specimen is provided. Some tests require voiding at specified times.

7. Place each specimen into the appropriately labeled container. For some tests each specimen is not kept separately but is poured into a large bottle in the laboratory refrigerator. Note assessment data for each specimen, if indicated for that.

8. If the outside of the specimen container is contaminated with urine, clean it with soap and water.

   Rationale Cleaning prevents the transfer of microorganisms to others.

9. Ensure that each specimen is refrigerated throughout the timed collection period. If not refrigerated, specimens are often kept on ice.

   Rationale Refrigeration or other form of cooling prevents bacterial decomposition of the urine.

10. Ask the client to provide the last specimen 5–10 minutes before the end of the collection period.

11. Assess the color, odor, and clarity of the client's urine.

12. Inform the client that the test is completed.

13. Remove the alert signs and specimen equipment from the client's unit and bathroom.

14. Document completion of the specimen collection on the client's chart. Include the date and specific time. In addition, if indicated for the specific test, note the time each urine specimen was collected, the volume of each specimen, the appearance of the urine, and other relevant data such as fluid intake or restrictions.

PROCEDURE 41–10   **Obtaining a Urine Specimen from a Retention Catheter**

Urine is aspirated from catheters using a sterile syringe and needle. When self-sealing rubber catheters are used, the needle is inserted just above the place where the catheter is attached to the drainage tubing. The area from which to obtain urine may be marked by a patch on the catheter. When plastic, silicone, or silastic catheters are used, the needle is inserted into the drainage tubing at a designated collection or sampling port. See Figure 41–1.

EQUIPMENT

- Disinfectant swab
- Sterile syringe (3 mL) and sterile 1-inch needle (#21–25 gauge)
- Sterile culture tube or unsterile bottle, depending on the purpose of the specimen
- Tubing clamp

INTERVENTION

1. Wipe the area where the needle will be inserted (collection port) with a disinfectant swab. The site should be remote from the tube leading to the balloon to avoid puncturing this tube.

   Rationale   Disinfecting the needle insertion site removes or destroys any microorganisms on the surface of the catheter, thereby avoiding contamination of the needle and the entrance of microorganisms into the catheter.

2. Insert the needle at a 30–45° angle.

   Rationale   This angle of entrance facilitates self-sealing of the rubber.

3. If urine is not readily available, elevate the tubing slightly to return urine to the area or clamp the tubing for 15 minutes.

4. Withdraw the required amount of urine, eg, 3 mL.

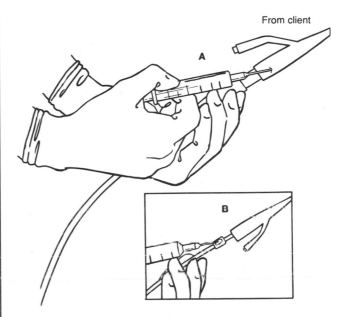

From client

Figure 41–1
Obtaining a urine specimen from a retention catheter: **A**, from a specific area, sometimes designated by a patch, near the end of the catheter; **B**, from a drainage port in the tubing.

5. Transfer the urine to the specimen container. Make sure the needle does not touch the outside of the container, if a sterile culture tube is used.

6. Cap and label the container and send the urine to the laboratory.

7. If the tubing was clamped, unclamp it.

   Rationale   Failure to unclamp the tubing may result in a distended bladder and discomfort for the client.

8. Document collection of the specimen and any pertinent observations of the urine on the appropriate records.

PROCEDURE 41–11 **Testing Urine for Specific Gravity, pH, Glucose, Ketones, and Occult Blood**

Specific Gravity

The specific gravity is the weight or degree of concentration of a substance compared with that of an equal volume of another (such as distilled water), which is taken as a standard. The specific gravity of distilled water is 1.00 g/mL (in other words, 1 mL of water weighs 1 g). The specific gravity of urine can be measured by a urinometer (hydrometer) calibrated in units of 0.001. The instrument is placed in a glass cylinder containing the urine. The scale on the urinometer progresses from 1.000 at the top to 1.060 at the bottom. The specific gravity of urine is normally about 1.010 to 1.025 g/mL. A low specific gravity in adults is often the result of overhydration or a disease that affects the kidneys' ability to concentrate solutes in the urine; in infants it is the result of immature kidneys, which are unable to concentrate urine. A high specific gravity is often the result of dehydration or a disease that increases water reabsorption by the kidneys, causing concentrated urine. False positive results are caused by drugs such as dextran and by radiopaque materials used in x-ray examinations of the urinary tract.

pH

The pH is a measurement of the concentration of hydrogen ions, which indicates the acidity or alkalinity of a substance. Discrete measurements of pH are made on a scale of 1–14, in which the value 7 is neutral, below 7 is acidic, and above 7 is alkaline (basic). Such quantitative measurements, however, are conducted in the agency laboratory, where specific reactive agents are used. Less discrete measurements of urinary pH (ie, to determine whether the urine is acidic or alkaline) can be made using litmus paper.

Urine becomes increasingly acidic when increasing amounts of sodium and excess acid are retained in the body. Ingestion of various foods also affects urinary pH. A diet rich in animal protein, milk, and cranberry juice decreases the pH and produces an acid urine. A diet high in citrus fruits, most vegetables, and jams and jellies increases the pH and produces an alkaline urine.

Control of the urine pH is an important factor in certain medical therapies. For example, the formation of renal stones is partially dependent on the urinary pH; therefore, clients being treated for stones are often given diets or medications to alter the pH and prevent stone formation. Certain medications—eg, streptomycin, neomycin, and kanamycin—are more effective for treating urinary tract infections provided the urine is alkaline.

Presence of Glucose

Urine is tested for glucose to screen clients for diabetes mellitus or to follow the progress of a known diabetic. Normally, the amount of glucose in the urine is negligible, although individuals who have ingested large amounts of sugar may show small amounts of glucose in their urine.

Several commercial products are commonly used to test for the presence of glucose, eg, Clinitest tablets and Clinistix, Diastix, and Tes-Tape reagent strips. Each uses a color scale to measure the quantity of glucose in the urine, but the scales are not interchangeable from one product to the other. The scales grade the results as negative, trace, one plus (1 +, or +), two plus (2 +, or + +), three plus (3 +, or + + +), etc. Each grade reflects a specific percentage of glucose, which varies from one testing product to another. For example, a 2 + result from a Clinitest reaction indicates 75% glucose in the urine, whereas a 2 + result from a Tes-Tape strip indicates 25% glucose.

False readings can arise from medications a client is receiving, depending on the type of chemical product used to test the urine for glucose. For example, tetracycline and large doses of ascorbic acid and chloral hydrate can generate false positive results from Clinitest tablets. For this reason, many agencies stock more than one testing product. Nurses need to compare the medications a client is receiving with the literature about each product and choose the appropriate product for the test.

Presence of Ketone Bodies

Ketone bodies are products of incomplete fat metabolism and appear in the urine in instances of fasting, very low intake of carbohydrates, and uncontrolled diabetes mellitus. Usually, the urine is tested for ketone bodies at the same time it is tested for glucose. Tablets or reagent strips are used.

Presence of Occult Blood

Normal urine is free of blood. When blood is present, it may be clearly visible or not visible (occult). Commercial reagent strips are used to test for occult blood in the urine.

EQUIPMENT

For Specific Gravity

- A urinometer (hydrometer) and a glass cylinder for the urine
    or
  A spectrometer or refractometer

For Urine pH

- Litmus paper (red or blue)

For Glucose

- A reagent tablet or reagent test strip
- The appropriate color scale
- A clean test tube and a dropper, if a tablet is used

For Ketone Bodies

- A reagent tablet or test strip

For Occult Blood

- A reagent strip

INTERVENTION

Measuring Specific Gravity

1. If a controlled specimen is ordered, ask the client to withhold fluids for the specified time, eg, 8 to 12 hours. When routine specific gravity measurements are being taken (eg, for clients with burns), fluids are not withheld.

2. To measure with a urinometer:
   a. Don gloves and pour at least 20 mL of a fresh urine sample in the glass cylinder, or fill the cylinder three-quarters full.
   b. Allow the specimen to come to room temperature—about 22 C or 72 F.
      Rationale   Most urinometers are calibrated for this temperature.
   c. Place the urinometer into the cylinder and give it a gentle spin to prevent it from adhering to the sides of the cylinder.

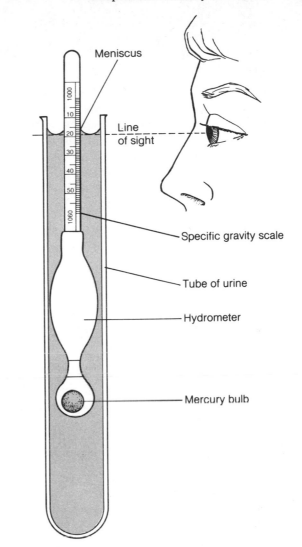

Figure 41–2

   d. Hold the urinometer at eye level, and read the measurement at the base of the meniscus at the surface of the urine. See Figure 41–2.
      Rationale   The concentration of the urine affects the degree to which the urinometer will float. The depth to which it sinks indicates the specific gravity.

3. To measure with a spectrometer or refractometer:
   a. Be sure to follow the manufacturer's directions.
   b. Don gloves and place one or two drops of urine on the slide.
   c. Turn on the instrument light, and look into the instrument. The specific gravity will appear on a scope.
   d. Write down the number, then turn off the instrument.
   e. Remove the urine with a damp towel or gauze.

Measuring pH

4. Put on a glove and dip a strip of either red or blue litmus paper into the urine specimen.

5. Observe the color of the litmus paper, and compare it to a standardized color chart on the bottle. The blue litmus paper, more commonly used, remains blue if the urine is alkaline and turns red if it is acidic. The red litmus paper remains red in the presence of acidic urine and turns blue if the urine is alkaline. Whichever litmus strip is used, red always indicates acidic urine and blue always indicates alkaline urine.

Testing for Glucose

6. Obtain a freshly voided specimen. Most agencies require a *second-voided specimen:* Ask the client to void, and in 30 minutes ask him or her to void again, providing a specimen for the test this time.

   Rationale A second-voided specimen more accurately reflects the present condition of the body. Urine that has accumulated in the bladder, eg, overnight, reflects the condition of the body at the time the urine was produced, eg, 0300 hours.

7. Select the appropriate equipment and testing product for the client. If Clinitest tablets are used, obtain a clean test tube and dropper.

8. To carry out the test, put on gloves and follow the directions specified by the manufacturer. If Clinitest tablets are used, be careful not to touch the bottom of the test tube because it becomes extremely hot when the tablet boils in the presence of urine and water.

9. Compare the results with the appropriate color chart, and record them on the client's chart. (Most agencies now record the findings as a percentage of glucose in the urine rather than as 2 + or 3 +.)

Testing for Ketone Bodies

10. Put on a glove and place one or two drops of urine on a reagent tablet (eg, an Acetest tablet), or dip a reagent test strip (eg, Ketostix) into the urine.

11. Observe and compare the results with the appropriate color chart to determine the quantity of ketones present.

12. Record the results in accordance with the product used and agency practice. The results may be graded as negative, small, moderate, or large amounts or as negative, positive, or strongly positive.

Testing for Occult Blood

13. Don a glove and dip the reagent strip (eg, Hemastix) into a sample of urine.

14. Compare the color change with a color chart in the same manner as with other reagent strips.

15. Discard the urine following the tests. Clean the equipment with soap and water. Remove gloves.

16. Document the results of the test on the client's record.

≋ Considerations for the Elderly

Many older adults have a lower specific gravity than younger adults because of decreased kidney tubular function. However, urine of elderly persons—like that of others—is most concentrated in the early morning.

A slight proteinuria (1 +) with the absence of sediment is not uncommon in older adults. A 24-hour urine collection for total protein is usually done if problems are suspected.

Glucosuria may occur in older persons due to a lower renal threshold for glucose. A glucose tolerance test is usually required to determine whether a disease process such as diabetes mellitus is the cause.

Freshly voided specimens of older adults may range between an acidic pH (eg, 4.6) and an alkaline pH (eg, 8), in contrast to younger adults, in whom freshly voided specimens are normally acidic.

PROCEDURE 41–12 Suprapubic Catheter Care

Two commonly used suprapubic catheters are the Cystocath and the Bonanno catheter. See Figure 41–3. These are narrow-lumen catheters. The Bonanno catheter has a curl at the distal end that prevents the catheter from being expelled by the bladder through the urethra. The Cystocath has a disc that holds the catheter in place on the abdominal wall; the Bonanno catheter has wings for that purpose. Attachments of the catheter to the drainage system tubing also vary: The Cystocath is joined with a stopcock; the Bonanno with a Luer-Lok adapter.

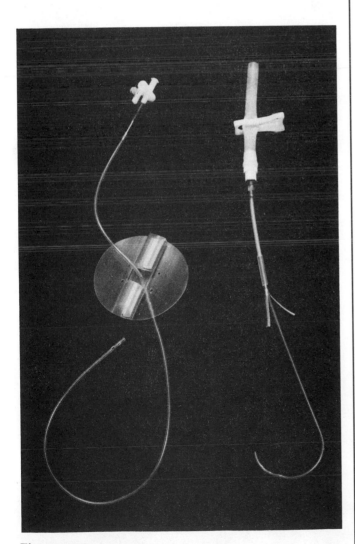

Figure 41–3
Two types of suprapubic catheters: Cystocath (left) and Bonanno (right).

Care of suprapubic catheters includes maintenance of a patent drainage system, skin care around the insertion site, periodic clamping of the catheter preparatory to removing it, and measurement of residual urine. The physician's order about management of the catheter is followed. Orders generally include leaving the catheter open to drainage for 48–72 hours, then clamping the catheter for 3- to 4-hour periods during the day until the client can void satisfactory amounts. Satisfactory voiding is determined by measuring the client's residual urine after voiding.

EQUIPMENT

For maintaining drainage:

- A sterile syringe (30–50 mL) with a #22 gauge needle (optional)
- Sterile saline solution or urinary irrigant (optional)
- Sterile alcohol swabs or povidone-iodine applicators

For a dressing change:

- A sterile dressing set containing:
  - 4 × 4 gauzes
  - Precut 4 × 4 drain sponges (eg, Telfa pads)
  - Povidone-iodine or hydrogen peroxide solution
  - Applicator swabs
  - A container for the solution
  - Povidone-iodine ointment
  - Forceps
  - Gloves
  - Nonallergenic tape
- A moisture-resistant line-saver pad
- A moisture-resistant bag for the soiled dressing

For removal of the catheter:

- A 3-mL syringe with a #22 gauge needle if a urine specimen is required
- Alcohol wipes
- A sterile dressing set with suture scissors

- 2 × 2 gauzes
- An Elastoplast bandage
- A moisture-resistant bag
- Gloves

INTERVENTION

1. Assess
   a. Color, consistency, clarity, and amount of urine drained. Assess hourly for the first 24 hours of observation and then at least three times daily.
   b. Fluid intake, to ensure it is adequate to maintain a satisfactory urine output.
   c. Bladder discomfort. Bladder spasms may occur during the first 24–48 hours. Spasms are identified by the presence of intermittent pain that does not affect the amount of urinary output.
   d. Indications of an obstruction in the drainage system. Obstruction is identified by distention and tenderness of the bladder (assessed by palpation), feelings of fullness, pubic pain, and a reduction in urinary output.
   e. Amount of residual urine after voiding. See earlier discussion.
   f. Redness and discharge at the skin around the insertion site.
   g. Vital signs, to compare to baseline data.

Maintaining the Catheter

2. Make sure the catheter and drainage tubes are securely connected. Tape these connections to avoid separation of the tubes.

3. If the catheter is not connected to drainage:
   a. Connect the catheter to a closed urinary drainage bag, maintaining the sterility of the ends of the tubes.
   b. Don gloves and initiate drainage by removing all air from the tubing. To remove air, clean the soft rubber connecting tubing of a Bonanno catheter or the marked injection port on the stopcock of the Cystocath with an alcohol swab or povidone-iodine applicator, insert a sterile syringe with a #22 gauge needle, pull back on the plunger, and aspirate until urine flows past the Luer-Lok connection (see Figure 41–4) or the stopcock. Make sure the Cystocath stopcock arrow is turned toward the collection bag and is open for drainage.

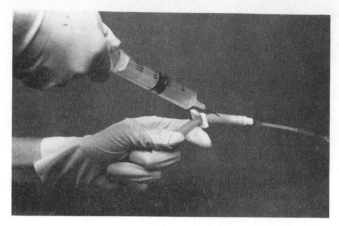

Figure 41–4

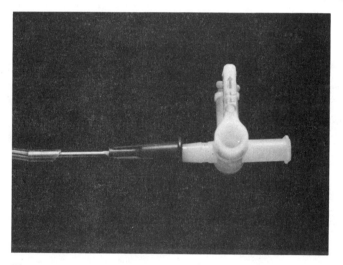

Figure 41–5

Rationale The catheter drains by siphonage. Removing the air creates a mild suction.

4. Ensure that the tubing is not kinked, that it runs straight up from the collection bag, and that excess tubing is coiled appropriately and taped to the client's abdomen or leg.

5. Make sure the Cystocath stopcock arrow is turned toward the part of the system to be turned off:
   a. For urine to drain, turn the arrow toward the rubber injection port on the stopcock. See Figure 41–5.
   b. For irrigating the catheter, turn the arrow toward the drainage bag so that fluid will flow into the client's bladder and not the bag. See Figure 41–6.
   c. For clamping the catheter, turn the arrow toward the catheter insertion site. See Figure 41–7.

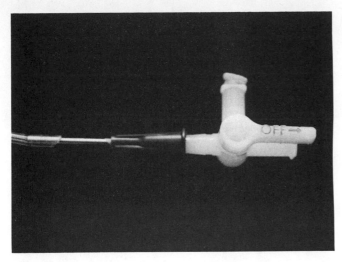

Figure 41–6

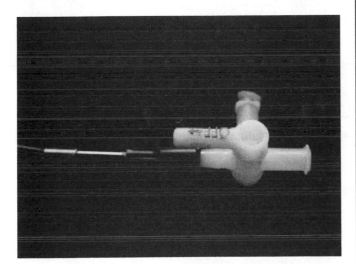

Figure 41–7

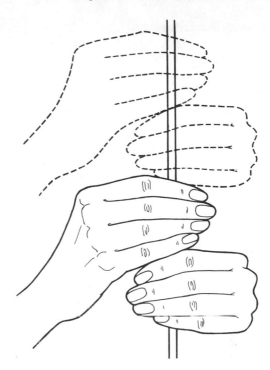

Figure 41–8

6. If urine does not drain well, implement the following steps in order:
   a. Have the client turn from side to side.

   Rationale Movement may dislodge obstruction of the tip of the catheter by the bladder wall.

   b. Milk the catheter tubing from the insertion site toward the drainage bag. See Figure 41–8.

   Rationale This can dislodge clots or sediment.

   c. As a last alternative and only if there is an order to irrigate the tubing:
   - Fill a sterile syringe with sterile normal saline or other urinary irrigant supplied by the agency, and attach a #22 needle, maintaining sterility.

- Clean the injection port of the catheter with an alcohol swab or povidone-iodine applicator.
- Insert the #22 needle and syringe as in step 3b.
- Slowly inject 30 mL of the irrigant.
- Observe the return flow of fluid by gravity.
- If fluid does not return, aspirate one-half the irrigant to dislodge a blood clot.
- Remove the needle.
- If a stopcock is present, turn the arrow toward the rubber injection site.

  Rationale This allows urine to drain from the catheter into the drainage bag.

   d. If the above actions fail:
   - Disconnect the catheter from the tubing, using strict surgical aseptic technique.
   - Clean the end of the catheter with an alcohol swab or povidone-iodine applicator.
   - Insert the syringe, filled with irrigant and without the needle, into the end of the catheter.
   - Instill the solution to irrigate the catheter, and then aspirate the clot.
   - Again clean the end of the catheter with the alcohol or iodine.
   - Reconnect the catheter to the drainage tubing.

Changing the Dressing

7. Assist the client to lie on the side opposite the drainage tube.

   Rationale This position exposes the tube more clearly.

8. Place the moisture-resistant pad under the client's hip below the drain.

9. Open the sterile dressing kit. Open the waste bag, roll its top edges outward, and place it away from the sterile field.

   Rationale Rolling the edges outward keeps the top of the bag open for use. Placing it away from the sterile field prevents contamination of the sterile field.

10. Carefully remove the tape from the suprapubic tube dressing. Using forceps, remove the soiled dressings, and discard them in the bag. A Cystocath may or may not have a dressing over the disc.

    Rationale Forceps are used to keep the nurse's hands clean.

11. When removing the tape and dressings, be careful not to jar the catheter.

    Rationale Jarring the catheter can cause bladder spasms.

12. Don sterile gloves.

13. Clean the catheter insertion site, using the sterile forceps.

    Rationale Forceps keep the gloves sterile for handling the dressings.

    a. Clean around the catheter insertion site as you would clean any surgical drain, moving from the insertion site outward. See Figure 41–9. Use a new swab for each wipe.

       Rationale Moving from the insertion site outward prevents wiping contaminants into the wound.

    b. Discard each used swab in the bag, being careful not to contaminate the forceps tips on the edge of the bag.

14. Apply a small amount of povidone-iodine ointment around the insertion site.

15. Place a precut 4 × 4 Telfa drain gauze around the suprapubic catheter over the insertion site.

    Rationale The Telfa dressing does not stick to the skin when it becomes soiled, and thus its removal is facilitated.

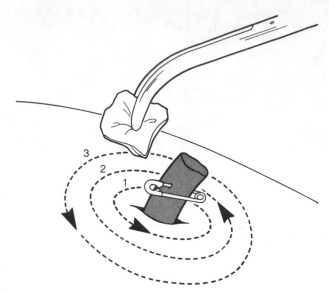

Figure 41–9

16. Place several uncut 4 × 4 gauzes over the Telfa gauze and catheter.

    Rationale These gauzes absorb drainage and support and stabilize the catheter.

17. Apply nonallergenic tape over the 4 × 4 gauzes to hold them in place.

18. Gently loop the catheter on the client's abdomen, and tape it in place.

    Rationale Looping prevents the catheter from pulling on the bladder.

Measuring Residual Urine

After the first few days of catheter insertion, the physician will order periodic catheter clamping, eg, every 3–4 hours, depending on the client's level of discomfort. The clamping will determine how well the client can void normally. After voiding, measure the residual urine.

19. When the catheter is clamped or closed by a stopcock:

    a. Have the client notify you of feelings of suprapubic discomfort or feelings of fullness.

       Rationale These feelings indicate a distended bladder, which can be confirmed by palpation.

    b. Ask the client to void normally, and measure the amount voided.

       Rationale Measurement indicates whether the client can void a satisfactory amount. Normally a person voids 150–350 mL of urine.

20. Empty the drainage bag attached to the catheter.
    Rationale This clears it for the residual urine measurement.

21. a. Unclamp the catheter or open the stopcock for about 5 minutes.

    b. Allow the residual urine to drain from the bladder through the catheter into the bag. After 5 minutes, measure it.
    Rationale Improper emptying of the bladder after voiding leaves larger than normal amounts of urine in the bladder. The physician may order removal of the catheter when the amount of residual urine is 100 mL or less.

    c. Following the first clamping period or as ordered, obtain a sterile specimen of the residual urine from the emptying spout of the bag.
    Rationale A sterile specimen of the first residual urine sample is often ordered for culture and sensitivity, to ensure that the urine and the bladder are free of microorganisms.

22. Ensure that the client's fluid intake is satisfactory, eg, 3000 mL/day or as ordered by the physician.

23. Record the procedure and your assessments on the appropriate records.

Sample Recording

Date	Time	Notes
6/7/89	1400	SP catheter draining well. Urine slightly pink. SP dressing dry and intact. ————
6/8/89	0600	SP catheter clamped. ————
	0900	Tolerated SP clamping for 3-hr period. Voided 90 mL urine. Residual urine 240 mL. Dressing changed. Small amount serosanguineous drainage. Insertion site appears clean. ———— ————————Sally M. Sharp, RN

Removing the Catheter

24. Using sterile technique and sterile gloves, remove the dressing, and dispose of it in the moisture-resistant bag. The Cystocath may or may not have a dressing over the disc.

25. Loosen the Cystocath disc.

26. Inspect the insertion site, and remove any sutures. (For removing sutures, see Procedure 45–7 in *Introduction to Nursing*.)

27. Remove the catheter with a steady, continuous pull.

28. Apply pressure over the insertion site with gauze squares.

29. Clean the site with antiseptic solution or swabs. Apply povidone-iodine ointment and an Elastoplast bandage.

URINARY DIVERSION OSTOMIES

There are four main types of urinary diversion ostomies:

1. Cutaneous ureterostomy

2. Ileal conduit

3. Vesicostomy

4. Ureterosigmoidostomy or ureteroileosigmoidostomy

Permanent urinary diversion stomas are indicated for any condition that requires a total cystectomy, eg, cancer of the bladder. Temporary urinary diversion stomas are indicated for any condition requiring partial cystectomy, eg, trauma to the lower urinary tract, or severe chronic urinary tract infections.

URETEROSTOMY

In cutaneous ureterostomy, the ureters are diverted to the abdominal wall or flank, and a ureteral stoma is formed. Ureterostomies are small compared to colostomies (about 0.5 mm or 1/4 inch in diameter) and drain continuously. They may involve the right or left ureter (*unilateral ureterostomy*, Figure 41–10, *A*) or both ureters (*bilateral ureterostomy*, Figure 41–10, *B*), in which case each one is covered by a separate appliance, unless they are placed close to each other.

Variations of the bilateral ureterostomy include:

1. The *double-barreled ureterostomy*, in which both ureters are brought to the skin surface to form side-by-side stomas. See Figure 41–10, *C*.

2. The *loop ureterostomy*, in which the ureters are looped out to the skin surface of each flank to form the stomas. See Figure 41–10, *D*.

3. The *transureteroureterostomy*, in which one ureter is first connected to the other, and then the receiving ureter is brought to the skin surface to form a stoma. See Figure 41–10, *E*.

ILEAL CONDUIT

The ileal (ileo) conduit is also referred to as *ileal (ileo) loop, ileal (ileo) bladder, ureteroileostomy,* or *Bricker's loop.* See Figure 41–11. In this procedure, a segment of the ileum is removed, and the intestinal ends are reattached. One end of the portion removed is closed with sutures to create an ileal pouch, and the other end is brought out through the abdominal wall

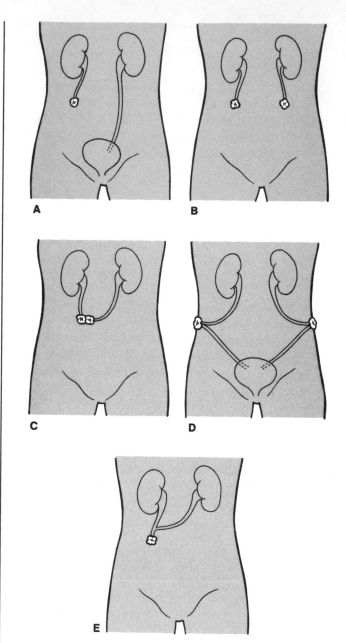

Figure 41–10
Five types of ureterostomies: **A,** right unilateral ureterostomy; **B,** bilateral ureterostomy; **C,** double-barreled ureterostomy; **D,** flank loop ureterostomy; **E,** transureteroureterostomy.

to create a stoma. The ureters are implanted into the ileal pouch, and the bladder is usually removed. The advantages of this procedure over ureterostomies are that the ileal stoma is larger and more readily fitted with an appliance; there is less chance of an ascending kidney infection, since the mucous membrane lining of the ileum acts as a barrier to microorganisms; and the stoma is less likely to stenose, a major

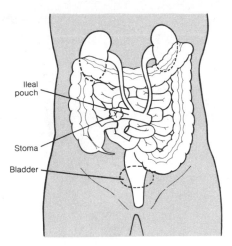

Figure 41–11
An ileal conduit.

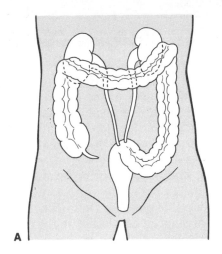

A

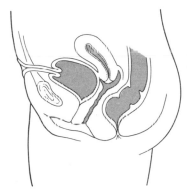

Figure 41–12
A continent vesicostomy.

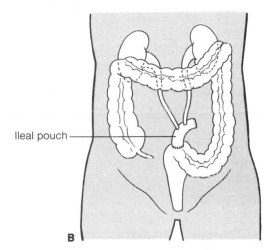

B

Figure 41–13
A, Ureterosigmoidostomy; **B,** ureteroileosigmoidostomy.

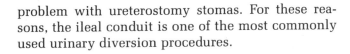

problem with ureterostomy stomas. For these reasons, the ileal conduit is one of the most commonly used urinary diversion procedures.

VESICOSTOMY

In vesicostomy, the anterior wall of the bladder is sutured to the abdominal wall, and a stoma is formed from the bladder wall. The urethral neck is sutured closed so that urine from the bladder empties directly through the stoma. To provide urinary control, a *continent vesicostomy* is usually performed. See Figure 41–12. In this procedure a tube is formed from part of the bladder wall. A stoma is formed at one end of the tube. A nipplelike valve is created from the bladder wall at the internal end. Urine drains through this type of vesicostomy only after a catheter is inserted through the stoma into the bladder pouch.

URETEROSIGMOIDOSTOMY

Ureterosigmoidostomy and ureteroileosigmoidostomy are two urinary diversion procedures that result in urine being excreted through the rectum. In ureterosigmoidostomy, the more common procedure, the ureters are implanted into the sigmoid colon. See Figure 41–13, A. One major complication with this type of procedure is pyelonephritis (infection of the kidney pelvis) from reflux of fecal material and intestinal microorganisms into the ureters and kidney pelvis. In ureteroileosigmoidostomy, a segment of the ileum is resected and connected to the sigmoid colon. The ureters are then implanted into this ileal pouch. See Figure 41–13, B. This procedure is thought to reduce the incidence of pyelonephritis. In both of these procedures, urine mixes with fecal material, resulting in very liquid stools and possible anal leakage of urine.

PROCEDURE 41–13 **Changing a Urinary Diversion Ostomy Appliance**

Various types of vinyl urinary stoma appliances are available (see Figure 41–14). The disposable one-piece pouch may be attached either to a nonallergenic adhesive-backed faceplate, which may or may not be precut, or to a semipermeable skin barrier, which is permeable to vapor and oxygen but impermeable to liquid. The latter attachment maintains skin integrity more effectively. Reusable pouches have opaque faceplates, which may or may not be attached to the pouch. Some have belt attachments, and one type has an adaptable insert that can be adjusted to stoma size. The enterostomal therapy nurse selects the pouch that best suits the client by considering the type of ostomy, the stoma location and shape, and the peristomal skin surface, as well as the client's body size and contour, physical and mental abilities, skin allergies, financial status, and life-style.

Generally, a urinary diversion appliance adheres to the skin for 2–5 days. They are usually changed twice a week. The nurse's responsibilities include stoma and peristomal care.

EQUIPMENT

If a commercially prepared stoma care kit is not available, the following supplies need to be assembled:

- Ostomy pouch with adhesive-backed faceplate
- Ostomy pouch belt (optional)
- Graduated pitcher or receptacle for the urine
- Basin filled with warm water, soap (optional), cotton balls, and towel
- Gauze pads
- Skin barrier (Skin Prep liquid or wipes or similar product, eg, Stomahesive or ready-made wafer-type or disc-type barrier) for the peristomal skin
- Stoma measuring guide
- Adhesive solvent in the form of presaturated sponges or liquid (optional)
- Adhesive cement (optional) for reusable pouches if double-faced adhesive disc is not used
- Scissors or electric razor
- Waterproof bag for the soiled appliance
- Gloves for the nurse

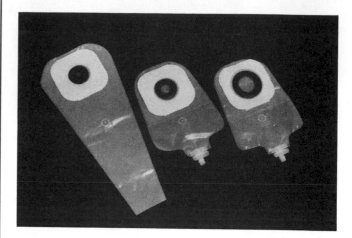

Figure 41–14
Examples of urinary appliances used for management of urinary diversion ostomies.

INTERVENTION

1. Obtain baseline assessment data.

2. Communicate acceptance and support of the client throughout the technique.

   Rationale This procedure often evokes negative emotional and psychologic responses from people.

3. Assist the client to a supine position in bed or to stand if able.

   Rationale A back-lying or standing position helps to separate abdominal skin folds that interfere with appliance application.

4. Unfasten the belt if one is being worn.

5. Don gloves.

6. Empty the urine from the pouch, when it is one-third to one-half full, into the graduated receptacle. It may be necessary to detach the pouch from a collection bag and tubing if the pouch is attached to a drainage system during the night. Pouches are often attached to a drainage system during the night to prevent accumulation and stagnation of urine in the appliance.

   Rationale The pouch is emptied when only one-third to one-half full because the weight of more urine may loosen the adhesive faceplate seal and separate the appliance from the skin.

7. Remove the appliance. Apply solvent, if needed, and peel the bag off slowly while holding the skin taut. Avoid touching the stoma with adhesive solvent.

   Rationale Holding the skin taut minimizes client discomfort and prevents skin abrasion. Adhesive solvent is irritating and may burn the stoma.

8. Discard a disposable appliance in a waterproof bag. If the appliance is reusable, wash it with lukewarm water and soap, and then air dry it to prevent it from becoming brittle.

9. Using cotton balls, carefully wash the peristomal skin with warm water and soap, if needed, and thoroughly rinse the soap from the area.

   Rationale Washing the area will remove stagnant urine, which has a strong odor. The oily residue of soap can prevent proper adherence of the appliance.

10. Dry the area thoroughly by patting with a towel or with cotton balls.

    Rationale Excessive rubbing can abrade the skin.

11. Assess the stoma and peristomal skin.

12. Place a gauze pad over the stoma, and change it as needed.

    Rationale The gauze pad will absorb the constant seepage of urine and prevent it from contacting the skin.

13. Remove excessive peristomal skin hair using scissors or an electric razor. Do not use a straight-edged razor.

    Rationale This will prevent discomfort and irritation of the hair follicles when the appliance is removed. It is easy to inadvertently damage the skin with a straight-edged razor.

Applying the Skin Barrier (Peristomal Seal)

14. If using Skin Prep liquid or wipes or other similar product:
    a. Cover the stoma with a gauze pad to avoid getting the Skin Prep on the stoma.
    b. Either wipe the Skin Prep evenly around the peristomal skin, or use an applicator to apply a thin layer of the liquid plastic coating to the area.
    c. Allow the Skin Prep to dry until it no longer feels tacky.

15. If using a wafer- or disc-type barrier, read the manufacturer's directions as well as the steps below. (Note that the karaya ring seal, although

effective in protecting the skin, is less effective with urinary ostomies than with bowel ostomies because urine tends to melt the product.)
    a. Use the stoma measuring guide to measure the size of the stoma.
    b. Trace a circle on the backing of the skin barrier the same size as the stomal opening.
    c. Make a template of the stoma pattern.
       Rationale A template aids other nurses and the client with future appliance changes.
    d. Cut out the traced stoma pattern to make an opening in the skin barrier.
    e. Remove the backing on one side of the skin barrier to expose the sticky adhesive.
    f. Attach the skin barrier to the faceplate of the ostomy appliance when it is prepared.
       Rationale Assembling the skin barrier and the appliance before application enhances the speed of application, an important consideration for constantly draining urostomies.

Preparing the Clean Appliance

16. To prepare a disposable pouch with adhesive square:
    a. If the appliance does not have the precut opening, trace a circle no more than 2–3 mm (⅛ in.) larger than the stoma size on the appliance's adhesive square.
       Rationale The opening is made slightly larger than the stoma to prevent rubbing, cutting, or trauma to the stoma.
    b. Cut out the traced circle in the adhesive. Take care not to cut any portion of the pouch.
    c. Peel off the backing from the adhesive seal, and attach the seal to a disc-type skin barrier or, if a liquid product was used, to the client's peristomal skin.

17. To prepare a reusable pouch with faceplate attached:
    a. Depending on the type of appliance, apply either adhesive cement or a double-faced adhesive disc to the faceplate. Follow the manufacturer's directions.

18. To prepare a reusable pouch with detachable faceplate:
    a. Remove the protective paper strip from one side of the double-faced adhesive disc.
    b. Apply the sticky side of the disc to the back of the faceplate.

c. Remove the remaining protective paper strip from the other side of the adhesive disc.

d. Attach the faceplate to a disc-type skin barrier or, if a liquid product was used, to the client's peristomal skin.

Applying the Clean Appliance

19. For a disposable pouch:

   a. Remove the gauze pad over the stoma before applying the pouch.

   b. Gently press the adhesive backing onto the skin and smooth out any wrinkles, working from the stoma outward.

      Rationale Wrinkles allow seepage of urine, which can irritate the skin and soil clothing.

   c. Remove the air from the pouch.

      Rationale Removing the air helps the pouch lie flat against the abdomen.

   d. Attach the spout of the pouch to a urinary drainage system or cap the spout. Temporary disposable pouches are often attached to drainage systems.

20. For a resuable pouch with faceplate attached:

   a. Insert a coiled paper guidestrip into the faceplate opening. The strip should protrude slightly from the opening and expand to fit it.

      Rationale The guidestrip helps in centering the appliance over the stoma and prevents pressure or irritation to the stoma by the appliance.

   b. Using the guidestrip, center the faceplate over the stoma.

   c. Firmly press the adhesive seal to the peristomal skin. The guidestrip will fall into the pouch; commercially prepared guidestrips will dissolve in the pouch.

   d. Place a deodorant in the bag (optional).

   e. Close the spout of the pouch with the designated cap.

   f. Optional: Attach the pouch belt and fasten it around the client's waist. Wash a soiled belt with warm water and mild soap, rinse, and dry if needed.

21. For a reusable pouch with detachable faceplate:

   a. Press and hold the faceplate against the client's skin for a few minutes to enhance the seal.

   b. Press the adhesive around the circumference of the adhesive disc.

   c. Tape the faceplate to the client's abdomen using four or eight 7.5-cm (3-in.) strips of tape. Place the strips around the faceplate in a "picture-framing" manner, one strip down each side, one across the top, and one across the bottom. The additional four strips can be placed diagonally over the other tapes to enhance the seal.

   d. Stretch the opening on the back of the pouch, and position it over the base of the faceplate. Ease it over the faceplate flange.

   e. Place the lock ring between the pouch and the faceplate flange to secure the pouch against the faceplate.

   f. Close the spout of the pouch with the appropriate cap.

   g. Optional: Attach the pouch belt and fasten it around the client's waist.

22. Assess the amount, color, and consistency of the drainage; the condition of the skin; and the client's response to the technique in terms of fatigue, discomfort, behavior about the ostomy, and skills learned.

23. Document all assessments and interventions.

24. Adjust the client's teaching plan and nursing care plan as needed. Include on the teaching plan the equipment and procedure used.

   Rationale Learning to care for the ostomy is facilitated if procedures implemented by nurses are consistent.

25. The client will also need to learn self-care and ways to reduce odor. Use of deodorant tablets in the appliance, soaking a reusable pouch in dilute vinegar solution, a diet that makes the urine more acid, and drinking plenty of fluids all help to control odor.

   Rationale A high fluid intake dilutes the urine, making it less odorous. Ascorbic acid and cranberry juice increase the acidity of urine, which in turn inhibits bacterial action and odor. Information about ostomy clubs and other community services available should also be included.

OXYGENATION

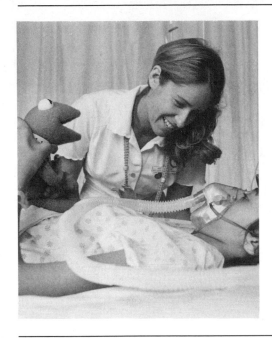

PROCEDURE 42–5 **Administering Oxygen by Face Tent**

Face tents can replace oxygen masks when masks are poorly tolerated by clients (eg, children). When a face tent is used alone to supply oxygen, the concentration of oxygen varies; therefore, it is often used in conjunction with a Venturi system.

EQUIPMENT

- An oxygen supply with a flowmeter
- A humidifier with sterile distilled water
- A face tent of the appropriate size (see Figure 42–1)

INTERVENTION

1. Follow Procedure 42–3, steps 1–4, in *Introduction to Nursing*. Encourage the client to handle the face tent.

2. Place the tent over the client's face, and secure the ties around the head.

3. Turn on the oxygen at the prescribed flow rate. Face tents can provide a 30–55% concentration of oxygen at 4–8 L/minute.

4. Assess the client's color, respirations, etc, and provide support for adjusting to the face tent.

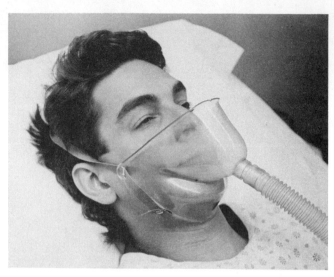

Figure 42–1
An oxygen face tent.

5. Follow Procedure 42–3, steps 10–13, in *Introduction to Nursing*.

6. Inspect the facial skin frequently for dampness or chafing, and dry and treat it as needed.

7. Document initiation of the therapy and all nursing assessments.

PROCEDURE 42–6   **Suctioning a Tracheostomy Tube**

Following a tracheostomy, the trachea and surrounding respiratory tissues are irritated and react by producing excessive secretions. Suctioning is necessary to remove these secretions and maintain a patent airway. The frequency of suctioning depends on the client's health and how recently the tracheostomy was done.

When suctioning a tracheostomy, use sterile technique to prevent infection of the respiratory tract.

EQUIPMENT

- Suction equipment, including a collection receptacle. The agency may have wall suction at the bedside, or it may use portable units.

- A sterile suction catheter. The diameter should be about half the inside diameter of the tracheostomy tube, to prevent hypoxia. Adults often require a #12 or 14 Fr. and children a #8 or 10 Fr. Some catheters have a thumb port on the side to control the suction.

- A Y-connector to join the catheter to the suction tubing if the catheter does not have a thumb port. One arm of the Y is then used to control the suction. A straight connector is used if the catheter has a thumb port.

- A container with sterile normal saline to lubricate and flush the catheter.

- A sterile 2- to 10-mL syringe and sterile normal saline without a bacteriostatic preservative for a tracheal lavage, if this is agency practice and/or is ordered. Lavage can liquefy tenacious secretions so that they are more easily suctioned out. The amount used is generally 0.5–1 mL for infants, 2 mL for children, and 2–5 mL for adults.

- Sterile gloves.

- A moisture-resistant bag in which to discard the disposable catheter and gloves.

- A sterile towel to provide an additional sterile area (optional).

- An oxygen source and flowmeter with a ventilator, or a manual resuscitator, eg, an Ambu or Laerdal bag.

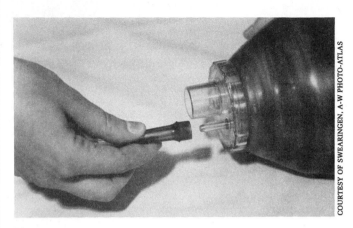

Figure 42–2

INTERVENTION

1. Obtain baseline assessment data.

2. Inform the client that suctioning usually causes intermittent coughing and that this assists in removing the secretions.

3. If permitted, place the client in semi-Fowler's position to promote deep breathing, maximum lung expansion, and productive coughing. Place an unconscious client in the supine position.
   Rationale   Deep breathing oxygenates the lungs, counteracts the hypoxic effects of suctioning, and may induce coughing. Coughing helps to loosen and move secretions.

4. Attach the resuscitation apparatus to the oxygen source. See Figure 42–2.

5. Open the sterile supplies in readiness for use.

6. Place the sterile towel, if used, across the client's chest below the tracheostomy.

7. Turn on the suction, and set the pressure in accordance with agency policy. Usually 100–120 mm Hg pressure is used for adults, and 50–75 mm Hg is used for infants and children.

8. Put on sterile gloves. Some agencies recommend putting a sterile glove on the dominant hand and an unsterile glove on the nondominant hand to protect the nurse.

9. Holding the catheter in the dominant hand and the connector in the nondominant hand, attach the catheter to the Y-connector or straight connector.

10. Using the sterile gloved hand, place the catheter tip in the sterile saline solution; using the thumb of the other hand, occlude the thumb control, and suction a small amount of sterile solution through the catheter.

    Rationale This determines that the suction equipment is working properly and lubricates the outside and the lumen of the catheter. Lubrication eases insertion and reduces tissue trauma during insertion. Lubricating the lumen helps prevent secretions from sticking to the inside of the catheter.

11. If the client does *not* have copious secretions, hyperventilate the lungs with a resuscitation bag before suctioning:

    a. Using your nondominant hand, turn on the oxygen to 12–15 L/minute.

    b. Attach the tracheostomy adapter of the resuscitator to the tracheostomy tube.

    c. Compress the Ambu or Laerdal bag as the client inhales, or every 5 seconds for an adult and every 3 seconds for an infant. This is best done by a second person who can use both hands to compress the bag, providing a greater inflation volume.

    d. Observe the rise and fall of the client's chest to assess the adequacy of the ventilation.
    or
    If the client has copious secretions, keep the regular wall-outlet oxygen delivery device on, and increase the liter flow for a few minutes before suctioning.

    Rationale Hyperventilating a client who has copious secretions can force the secretions deeper into the respiratory tract.

12. Remove the oxygen device.

13. With your nondominant thumb off the suction port, quickly but gently insert the catheter into the trachea through the tracheostomy tube. See Figure 42–3. Insert the catheter about 10–12.5 cm (4–5 in.) or until the client coughs.

    Rationale To prevent tissue trauma and oxygen loss, suction is not applied during insertion of the catheter.

14. Apply suction for 5–10 seconds by placing the nondominant thumb over the thumb port. Rotate

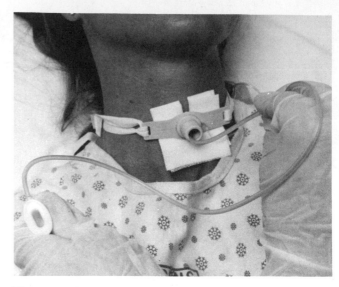

Figure 42–3

the catheter by rolling it between your thumb and forefinger while slowly withdrawing it.

Rationale Suction time is restricted to 10 seconds or less to minimize oxygen loss. Rotating the catheter as it is withdrawn prevents tissue trauma by minimizing the suction time against any part of the trachea.

15. Withdraw the catheter completely, and release the suction.

16. If secretions are thick, flush the catheter in the sterile solution, and insert 3–5 mL of sterile saline solution through the tracheostomy tube into the trachea. Then suction.

17. Reapply the source of supplementary oxygen if required. Observe the client's respirations and skin color, and allow the person to rest for a few minutes.

18. Encourage the client to breathe deeply and cough. Repeat steps 11–15 until the air passage is clear and the breathing is relatively effortless and quiet. Do not suction for more than 3–5 minutes in total.

    Rationale Suctioning too long can decrease the client's oxygen supply.

19. If agency policy indicates, and if the client's health warrants it, hyperoxygenate the lungs for a few minutes after each suction attempt and on completion of the suctioning procedure.

    Rationale This relieves hypoxia that may be created by suctioning.

20. Turn off the suction, and disconnect the catheter from the suction tubing.

21. Holding the catheter in your gloved hand, grasp the cuff of the glove with your other hand, and peel the glove off so that it turns inside out over the catheter.

22. Discard the glove and the catheter in the moisture-resistant bag.

23. Provide oral or nasal hygiene.

24. Inspect the amount of secretions obtained by suction, including the color, odor, and thickness.

25. Assist the client to a comfortable, safe position that aids breathing. If the person is conscious, a semi-Fowler's position is frequently indicated. If the person is unconscious, Sims' position can assist the drainage of secretions from the mouth.

26. Replenish the sterile fluid and supplies so that the suction is ready to be used again.

    Rationale Clients who require suctioning often require it quickly, so it is essential to leave the equipment at the bedside ready for use.

27. Document the suctioning, including the amount and description of suction returns, the amount of sterile saline instilled, and any other assessments.

PROCEDURE 42–7 **Assisting Clients with Intermittent Positive Pressure Breathing**

Intermittent positive pressure breathing (IPPB) is the delivery of air or oxygen into the lungs at positive (above atmospheric) pressure during inspiration and automatic release of the pressure when the predetermined positive pressure level is reached in the air passages. The result is that expiration occurs passively. Some IPPB machines can exert pressure during expiration, and the abbreviations IPPB/I (inspiratory) and IPPB/E (expiratory) are sometimes used to differentiate the two methods. Generally, however, IPPB refers to positive pressure therapy administered during inspiration, a safer and more common practice.

Various IPPB machines are marketed. Two commonly used types are the Bird respirator and the Bennett respirator. Assembly and maintenance of respirators is usually done by respiratory therapists. The machine is connected to an oxygen supply and is equipped with an in-line humidifier, which must be filled with distilled water. The client breathes through a mouthpiece or a mask attached to the end of the respirator tubing. See Figure 42–4.

Usually, IPPB treatments are given by respiratory therapists or by nurses who have had special education. However, the general nurse needs to understand the reason for IPPB therapy and its principles, to assist clients as needed in the absence of special therapists. The nurse must also observe the client's progress and response to such therapy. This discussion is limited to IPPB therapy that is client-activated and given on an intermittent basis. Controlled or time-cycled continuous therapy is used for people unable to initiate inspiration. The breathing of such people is maintained entirely by machine.

IPPB treatments are administered for one or more of the following reasons:

- To increase the depth of respirations periodically and prevent accumulation of secretions that may result in infections or atelectasis

- To facilitate the clearing of bronchial secretions in clients who have difficulty coughing or inhaling deeply

- To provide moisture to the respiratory mucous membranes

- To administer aerosol medications

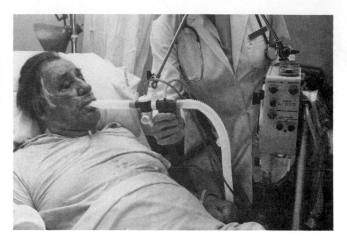

Figure 42–4
Intermittent positive pressure breathing (IPPB).

IPPB treatments are scheduled so that they do not conflict with meal hours, if possible. IPPB therapy is generally prescribed for five to six breaths hourly during waking hours. It should not be scheduled right before or after a meal, since it can induce nausea and a full stomach prevents maximum lung expansion.

THE BIRD RESPIRATOR

There are several types of Bird respirators; all are equipped with six basic controls (see Figure 42–5):

- The pressure control setting establishes the pressure that will be received at the height of an inspiration before the client enters the expiratory phase. It measures the pressure in centimeters of water pressure, from 0 to 60 cm. Usually, the pressure is started low, at 15 or 20 cm H_2O, and gradually increased as the client becomes accustomed to the machine.

- The flow rate control adjusts the inspiratory time and switches the ventilator from off to on. It is similar to a water tap: The more it is turned on, the faster the flow of gas. Low numbers on this dial indicate slow rates, and higher numbers indicate faster rates. Since the aim of therapy is usually to achieve deep respirations and transfer of gases deep

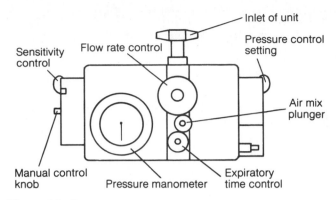

Figure 42–5
A schematic of the Bird respirator.

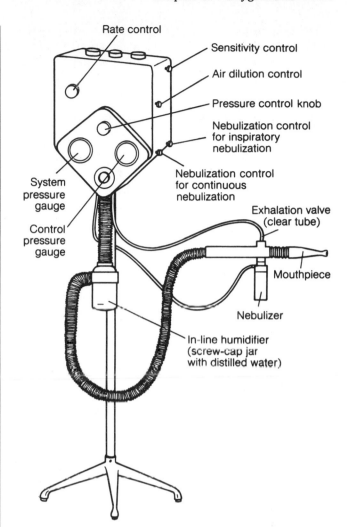

Figure 42–6
A schematic of the Bennett respirator.

into the alveoli, the flow rate is generally set at 10 or less to coincide with the client's inspiratory effort. Fast flow rates tend to flood only the upper respiratory tract. Effective flow rates can be assessed by observing the client's chest expansion during therapy.

- The air mix plunger determines the proportion of oxygen and air delivered to the client. It has two positions. When the plunger is pushed in, 100% of oxygen is delivered. When it is pulled out, a mixture of 40% oxygen and 60% air is delivered. These proportions cannot be varied as they can on more sophisticated respirators. Generally, the oxygen/air mixture is used.

- The sensitivity control adjusts the inspiratory effort required by the client to trigger or trip the machine (start the flow of gas). Once the machine is triggered, the pressure automatically builds to the peak pressure that was set by the pressure control knob. The smaller the number set on the sensitivity control, the higher the sensitivity (ie, the less effort required by the client to start the machine). People who are weak often require a high sensitivity control (low number setting) to start the machine, but people who need to be encouraged to breathe deeply should use a low sensitivity control (high number) that offers more resistance and requires more effort. The sensitivity control is usually set at 15 when starting therapy.

- The manual control knob, a pink knob or pin below the sensitivity control, can be pushed in manually to trigger the ventilator. It is mostly used to check respirator function before applying it to the client.

- The expiratory time control is turned to "off" for client-cycled IPPB. It is used only for people who are apneic or who require continuous assisted ventilation.

THE BENNETT RESPIRATOR

The Bennett respirator, shown in Figure 42–6, is different in appearance from the Bird respirator, but its operation is similar. The PR-1 model, which is frequently used, has many of the basic controls discussed for the Bird machine:

- The pressure control knob, capable of delivering 0–45 cm H_2O pressure, is rotated clockwise and generally set at 15–20 cm H_2O for adults or 10–12 cm H_2O for children. The initial pressure setting may be lower.

- The control pressure gauge records the pressure that is reached by turning the pressure control knob.

- The system pressure gauge records the pressure that is required by the client and should equal that measured by the control pressure gauge at the end of inspiration.

- The air dilution control is usually pushed in to allow for an air/oxygen mixture. When it is pulled out, 100% oxygen is delivered.

- The sensitivity control determines the amount of inspiratory effort required to start inspiration and is used only if the client has difficulty triggering the machine. Indications of difficulty are determined when people say they are sucking or drawing on the machine to no avail or when the system pressure gauge needle deflects to the negative side. In these instances the sensitivity control should be set higher so that less effort is required by the client to trigger the machine.

- The rate control regulates the rate of automatic cycling and is turned to the "off" position for client-cycled IPPB.

- The nebulization controls provide power to the side steam nebulizer to deliver aerosol medications. One knob sets the nebulizer for continuous therapy, the other for inspiratory nebulization. If a client is receiving a medicated treatment, the inspiration knob is generally turned one revolution to ensure adequate nebulization on inspiration. With the use of the continuous knob, the medication is delivered immediately upon inspiration.

EQUIPMENT

- An IPPB machine.

- A mouthpiece.

- A noseclip (optional).

- A mask (to be used only if a mouthpiece and a noseclip are not effective).

- A source of pressurized air and oxygen if the machine does not have an internal compression unit.

- Sterile normal saline solution or the prescribed aerosol medication, eg, 1% isoetharine hydrochloride (Bronkosol). Routine measured IPPB medication doses are commercially available in plastic ampules.

- A 3-mL syringe with a needle to prepare the medication or saline.

- A Wright respirometer (optional) and an exhaled volume collector.

- Tissues and a moistureproof waste bag or other container for expectorated secretions.

INTERVENTION

1. Verify the physician's orders and check whether aerosol medications are to be administered during therapy. Bronchodilators, mucolytics, or antibiotics may be ordered.

2. Explain that the therapy will assist the client to achieve deep lung expansion and will promote coughing and removal of secretions.

3. Assist the client to a Fowler's position in bed or to sit upright in a chair.

   Rationale These positions facilitate maximal lung expansion.

4. Obtain baseline assessment data.

5. Teach the client to breathe normally through the mouth by using the mouthpiece and refrain from breathing through the nose. Have the client practice breathing only through the mouthpiece prior to therapy. Ensure that the mouthpiece is completely sealed by the lips. Have the client use a noseclip if breathing only through the mouth is difficult.

   Rationale Mouth breathing and an airtight seal around the mouthpiece are essential for efficient operation of the IPPB system.

6. Adjust the pressure control setting on a Bird respirator or the pressure control knob on a Bennett respirator to 10–15 cm H_2O. See Figure 42–5 for a Bird respirator, Figure 42–6 for a Bennett respirator.

   Rationale This control sets the pressure that will be received at the height of an inspiration.

7. Fill the nebulizer with sterile saline or prescribed medication, reattach it, and set the nebulization control if necessary. See Figure 42–7. If a medication is used, prepare it before going to the client.

   Rationale Nebulization delivers prescribed medications and/or moisture to the respiratory mucous membranes. IPPB therapy must be given with medication or sterile saline in the nebulizer unless a mainstream humidifier is used. Air that is not moisturized dries the airways and impedes the mobilization of secretions.

8. Set the oxygen/air mix control as ordered. For a mixture of air and oxygen, pull the knob of a Bird

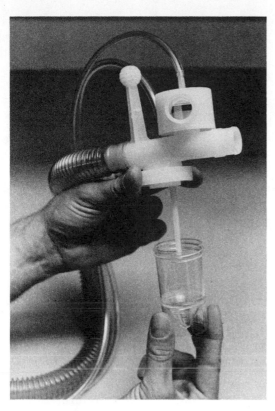

Figure 42-7

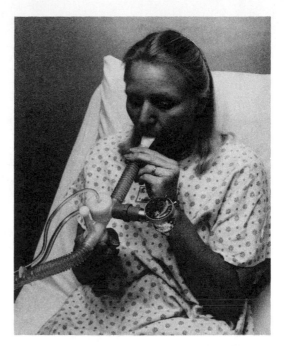

Figure 42-8

respirator out, push the knob of a Bennett respirator in.

9. Occlude the end of the tubing that will be attached to the mouthpiece, and manually cycle the machine to operate.

   Rationale This ensures that the system is airtight and that it cycles off at the preset pressure. If the desired pressure is not reached, the nurse needs to check for a leak in the system, eg, a disconnection in the nebulizer.

10. Attach the mouthpiece to the machine's tubing.

11. Have the client place the lips tightly around the mouthpiece, relax, and inhale deeply and slowly through the mouth as the machine cycles on.

    Rationale The machine will not start until the client breathes in.

12. Encourage the client to breathe in until the lungs are maximally inflated. Explain that the machine will cycle off when the preset pressure is met or when the client breathes out.

    Rationale By allowing the pressure to reach its peak before exhaling, maximal lung expansion is achieved when the appropriate pressure is set.

13. Optional: After full inspiration, have the client hold the breath for a few seconds.

    Rationale This provides greater distribution of oxygen, air, and nebulized particles.

14. Instruct the client to exhale normally in a relaxed and passive manner.

    Rationale Forced exhalation can increase small airway obstructions.

15. Observe the client for adequate chest expansion with each inhalation and for a relaxed, passive exhalation. Check that the needle gauges reach the preset pressure levels as the client inhales. See the pressure manometer in Figure 42-5 and the system pressure gauge in Figure 42-6.

    Rationale Although the degree of lung expansion can be observed visually, the gauges on the respirator provide more reliable measures. If the needle gauge on the respirator reaches the preset level during inhalation, the setting is usually satisfactory.
    or
    It is preferable to attach a Wright respirometer to the expiratory port of the IPPB manifold. See Figure 42-8. The Wright respirometer specifically measures the expired tidal volume and/or inspiratory capacity and indicates whether the client is receiving adequate deep lung inflations. Tidal volume is the volume of air inspired and expired

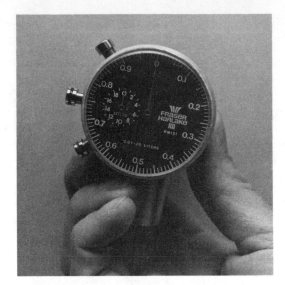

Figure 42–9

with a normal breath, about 500 mL. Inspiratory capacity is the maximum volume of air inspired after normal exhalation. The Wright respirometer usually has two dials: a large peripheral dial, which measures the volume from 0 to 100 L, and a smaller dial set inside, which measures tenths of a liter from 0 to 1 L. See Figure 42–9.

16. If there is inadequate or no deflection of the needle gauges:

    a. Check that the system is airtight. The client may not have sealed the lips around the mouthpiece adequately. If this is the case, decrease the pressure setting until the client feels comfortable, and then gradually increase the pressure. A noseclip may be necessary.

    b. Check that the client is relaxed. Perhaps the person is not breathing normally or is blowing back into the mouthpiece before the lungs are filled. If this is the case, encourage the client to breathe normally. Some clients have a tendency to force their breathing or to struggle with the apparatus. When advised not to force breaths, to relax, to breathe slowly, and to allow time for expiration (which takes longer than inspiration), people normally adjust to the therapy readily. Remind the client that he or she controls the machine: With each inhalation the machine starts; each time the client breathes out, the machine stops at peak inspiration. Extra effort by the client is not required.

    c. Check that the machine is triggering. Perhaps the client does not exert sufficient inspiratory effort to start the machine. In that case, adjust the sensitivity gauge to a lower number. If the needle deflection is negative, the client may be sucking, or using too much inspiratory effort, or the peak flow could be too low.

17. Monitor the client's blood pressure and pulse rate during the therapy, especially at the initial treatment. Stay with the person throughout the treatment. Stop the treatment and notify the physician if there is a sudden significant increase in pulse rate (20 or more beats per minute) or a sudden change in blood pressure (10 mm Hg or more). During subsequent IPPB sessions, blood pressure assessment is necessary only if the client has a history of cardiovascular disease, hypotension, or sensitivity to any medications given during therapy.

    Rationale Some bronchodilators, eg, isoproterenol and isoetharine, significantly increase the heart rate. IPPB therapy increases intrathoracic pressure and may cause a temporary decrease in cardiac output and venous return, indicated by hypotension, headache, and tachycardia.

18. If vital signs are stable, continue the IPPB therapy if indicated, until all the medication in the nebulizer is administered, or 15–20 minutes.

19. Following or during the therapy, encourage the client to expectorate respiratory secretions, as needed. Note the amount of sputum.

20. Auscultate the lung fields, and compare the pretherapy assessment. Note any improvement in aeration and absence of or diminished adventitious breath sounds, eg, rales, rhonchi, wheezes, or friction. Improvements may not be observable until 10–20 minutes after the therapy.

21. Clean the mouthpiece and nebulizer with sterile water, and dry them thoroughly. Store the mouthpiece in a plastic bag at the bedside or in accordance with agency policy. Generally, the mouthpiece is replaced every 24 hours for aseptic reasons.

22. Document the IPPB therapy, its duration, the medication administered, the pressure used, the volume achieved, the breath sounds and other assessments before and after the therapy, eg, the amount of sputum expectorated.

Sample Recording

Date	Time	Notes
9/2/89	1500	IPPB administered, 800-mL volume at 15 cm H_2O pressure with sterile normal saline nebulization for 15 min. Adventitious breath sounds absent 15 min. after treatment. BP 120/70, P 78, stable, before and after therapy. No secretions expectorated.————————Constance S. Boyd, RN

PROCEDURE 42–8 **Collecting a Sputum Specimen**

Sputum specimens ordered for culture and sensitivity are obtained to identify a specific microorganism and its drug sensitivities. Specimens for cytology often require serial collection of three early morning specimens and are tested to identify cancer in the lung and its specific cell type. Specimens for acid-fast bacillus (AFB), which also require serial collection (often for 3 consecutive days), are obtained to identify the presence of this organism, also known as the tubercle bacillus (TB). Some agencies use a special glass container when the presence of AFB is suspected.

EQUIPMENT

- A container with a cover for the sputum. These are often made of plastic.

- Disinfectant and swabs, or liquid soap and water, to clean the outside of the container, and paper towels to dry it.

- A completed label for the container, with identifying information about the client.

- A completed requisition to accompany the specimen to the laboratory.

- Mouthwash.

INTERVENTION

1. Inform the client about the need for the specimen and how to obtain one. If the client finds it painful to cough, eg, after abdominal surgery, demonstrate how to hold a pillow firmly against the affected area while coughing. This provides external support and decreases the discomfort. If the client needs to assume a postural drainage position to obtain the specimen, explain this, and arrange a time. In some instances pharyngeal suctioning may be required to obtain the specimen.

2. Make sure the client can expectorate the sputum directly into the sputum cup without allowing the sputum to contact the outside of the container. If nursing assistance is not required, leave the container with the client.

3. If nursing assistance is required, ask the client to hold the sputum cup on the outside, or hold it for a client who is not able. See Figure 42–10.

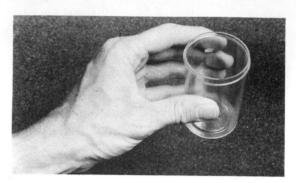

Figure 42–10

4. Ask the client to breathe deeply and then cough up 1–2 tbsp (15–30 mL, or 4–8 fluid drams). Some agencies may specify another amount.

5. Hold the sputum cup so the client can expectorate into it, making sure that the sputum does not come in contact with the outside of the container.
   Rationale Containing the sputum within the cup restricts the spread of microorganisms to others.

6. Assess the appearance and amount of sputum. The consistency of sputum can be described as liquid or thick. The color can be described as white, yellow, blood-tinged, green, or clear. The amount can be described as approximately 1 tsp or 1 tbsp.

7. Cover the container with the lid immediately after the sputum is in the container.
   Rationale Covering the container prevents the inadvertent spread of microorganisms to others.

8. Determine the respiration rate and note any abnormalities or difficulty breathing.

9. Assess the color of the client's skin and mucous membranes, especially any cyanosis, which can indicate impaired blood oxygenation.

10. Wipe the outside of the container with a disinfectant if the sputum has contacted the outside surface. Some agencies recommend washing the outside of all containers with liquid soap and water and then drying with a paper towel.

11. Place the completed label on the container.

12. Provide the client with mouthwash to rinse the mouth.
    Rationale This removes any unpleasant taste.

13. Arrange for the specimen and the completed laboratory requisition to be transported to the laboratory. Specimens that are taken for culture need to be sent directly to the laboratory, where they are placed in a bacteriologic refrigerator. If the specimen is to remain on the nursing unit, it needs to be refrigerated. When 24-hour specimens are collected, they may be sent to the laboratory once the container is about three-fourths full. Containers are only partly filled to ensure that the outside of the container is not in contact with the sputum. In some agencies the sputum specimens are kept in the specimen refrigerator in separate glass containers, which are numbered in the order in which they were taken. All the specimens collected during the 24-hour period are then sent to the laboratory.

14. Document collection of the sputum specimen on the client's chart. Include the color, consistency, and odor of the sputum, any measures needed to obtain the specimen (eg, postural drainage), the general amount of sputum produced, and any discomfort experienced by the client.

Sample Recording

Date	Time	Notes
6/21/89	0600	Sputum specimen sent to laboratory. Produced approximately 2 tbsp of green-yellow thick sputum. States has "sharp, knifelike pain" in right anterior lower chest when coughing. Sheila D. Wry, NS

Considerations for the Elderly

Ensure that older adults have sufficient fluid intake to maintain the effectiveness of the mucous membrane and cilia. Older adults may have difficulty in expectorating sputum due to decreased expansion of the lungs, decreased muscle strength in the thorax and diaphragm, and reduced cilia to remove mucus.

CHEST DRAINAGE SYSTEMS

Because the pleural cavity normally has negative pressure, any drainage system connected to it must be sealed, so that air or liquid cannot enter. See Figure 42–11. Such a drainage system is called a *water-sealed (underwater) drainage* or a *disposable pleural drainage system*. In water-sealed drainage, fluid in the bottom of the container prevents air from entering the chest tube and thus entering the pleural cavity. The system must be kept below the level of the client's chest, so that the fluid in the container is not drawn into the pleural cavity by gravity. It is also very important to maintain the patency of the tubing.

Drainage systems use three mechanisms to drain fluid and air from the pleural cavity: positive expiratory pressure, gravity, and suction. When the pleural cavity contains some air or fluid, a positive pressure develops during expiration. This positive pressure is abnormal, but it does help expel the air and to some extent fluid from the space. Gravity acts as an evacuation force when the tubing is placed so that it descends from the insertion site to the drainage receptacle. Suction is used in conjunction with the other two forces in some drainage systems.

There are several kinds of water-sealed drainage systems: one- and two-bottle gravity systems, two- and three-bottle suction systems, and disposable unit systems.

ONE-BOTTLE SYSTEMS

In a one-bottle system, a single receptacle both receives the fluid and/or air from the client and seals the system. See Figure 42–12. The client's air or fluid enters through the collection inlet, which terminates under sterile water, and air exits through the air vent. The fluid in this bottle then is a combination of fluid from the client and sterile water; it forms the water seal. The one-bottle system depends upon gravity and positive expiratory pressure for drainage.

TWO-BOTTLE SYSTEMS

A two-bottle system uses one bottle to receive the fluid or air from the client and the second bottle to create the water seal. See Figure 42–13. The client's air or fluid is received into bottle A. The air from bottle A is passed into bottle B. The air then exits from bottle B through the air vent. This system uses gravity and positive expiratory pressure for drainage.

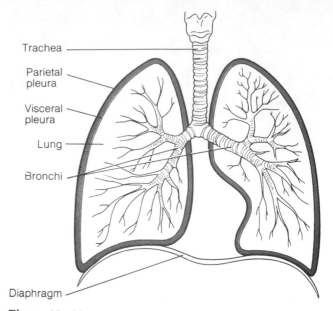

Figure 42–11
The pleural cavity is a potential space that lies between the visceral pleura and the parietal pleura. Chest tubes are inserted into this space.

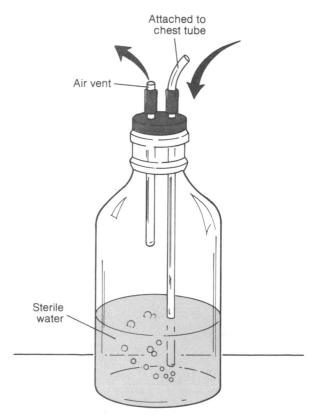

Figure 42–12
A one-bottle gravity water-sealed drainage system.

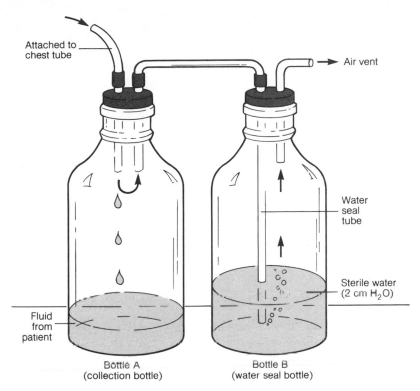

Attached to chest tube

Air vent

Water seal tube

Sterile water (2 cm H$_2$O)

Fluid from patient

Bottle A (collection bottle)

Bottle B (water seal bottle)

Figure 42–13
A two-bottle gravity water-sealed drainage system.

Another type of two-bottle system uses suction as well as positive expiratory pressure and gravity for drainage. See Figure 42–14. In this system, bottle A collects the fluid drainage from the client and creates the water seal. Bottle B is the suction-control bottle; the depth of the tube below the water level determines the amount of negative pressure provided (ie, the deeper the tube is submerged in the sterile water, the greater the vacuum).

THREE-BOTTLE SYSTEMS

The three-bottle system has a collection bottle (A), a water-seal bottle (B), and a suction-control bottle (C). See Figure 42–15. Fluid from the client collects in bottle A, which is connected to a tube in bottle B that terminates below the fluid level. Bottle B is then connected to bottle C by a short tube. Bottle C also has a manometer tube submerged in sterile water. The depth to which this tube is submerged determines the amount of suction exerted in the client's pleural cavity. The suction-control bottle has another inlet, for suction. This system uses positive expiratory pressure, gravity, and suction for drainage.

DISPOSABLE UNIT SYSTEMS

Disposable chest drainage systems are now more frequently used than the bottle drainage systems. Several types of disposable unit systems are available commercially. Two commonly seen are the Pleur-evac system and the Argyle system. The Pleur-evac system consists of three chambers. See Figure 42–16. Chamber A is the collection chamber. It receives fluid and/or air from the client and is divided into three subchambers. The client's fluid remains in this chamber, while air from the client passes on to chamber B, the water-seal chamber. This chamber is U-shaped, and air from the client passes through the water seal and exits at the suction outlet side of the U. Chamber C, the suction chamber, is also U-shaped. The height of the fluid in chamber C determines the amount of suction pressure exerted upon the client. Atmospheric air enters on the far left of this chamber, passes through the suction-control water, and joins the air from the client. These then pass into the suction outlet.

The Argyle double-seal system consists of four chambers. See Figure 42–17. Chamber A is a water-seal chamber with a manometer. Chamber B is the collection chamber. Chamber C is another water seal. Chamber D is for suction control. Normally the client's

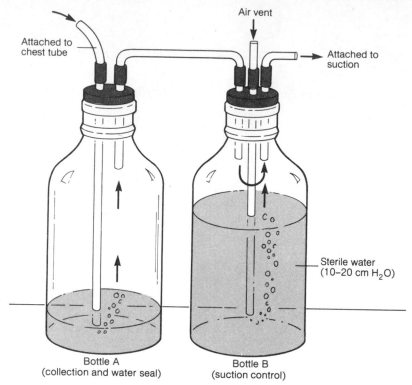

Attached to chest tube

Air vent

Attached to suction

Sterile water (10–20 cm H$_2$O)

Bottle A (collection and water seal)

Bottle B (suction control)

Figure 42–14
A two-bottle suction water-sealed drainage system.

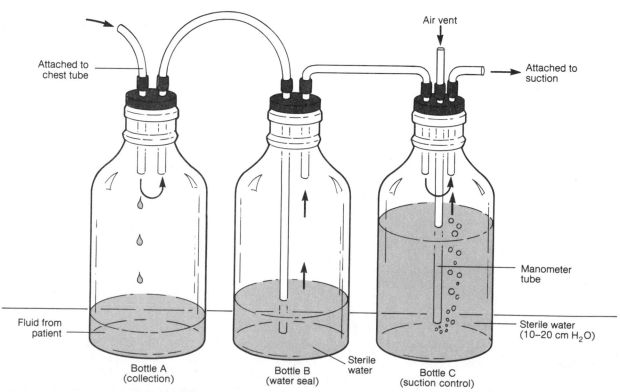

Attached to chest tube

Air vent

Attached to suction

Fluid from patient

Manometer tube

Sterile water

Sterile water (10–20 cm H$_2$O)

Bottle A (collection)

Bottle B (water seal)

Bottle C (suction control)

Figure 42–15
A three-bottle suction water-sealed drainage system.

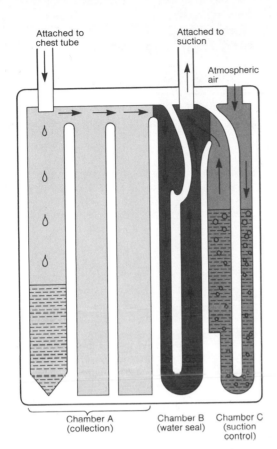

Figure 42–16
A Pleur-evac chest drainage system.

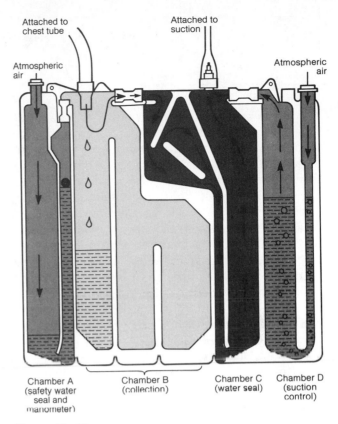

Figure 42–17
An Argyle chest drainage system.

air passes from chamber B into chamber C and to the suction source; however, if the suction becomes obstructed, the client's air can pass to chamber A and to the atmosphere. Chamber A thus serves as a safety vent.

PROCEDURE 42–9 **Assisting with the Insertion and Removal of a Chest Tube**

Chest tubes are inserted and removed by the physician with the nurse assisting. Both procedures require sterile technique and must be done without introducing air or microorganisms into the pleural cavity. After the insertion, an x-ray film is taken to confirm the position of the tube. Chest tubes are generally removed within 5–7 days. Before removal, the tube is clamped with two large, rubber-tipped clamps for 1–2 days to assess for signs of respiratory distress and to determine whether air or fluid remains in the pleural space. An x-ray film of the chest is generally taken 2 hours after tube clamping to determine full lung expansion. If the client develops signs of respiratory distress or the film indicates pneumothorax, the tube clamps are removed, and chest drainage is maintained. If neither occurs, the tube is removed. Another x-ray film of the chest is often taken after removal to confirm full lung expansion.

EQUIPMENT

For tube insertion:

- A sterile chest tube tray, which includes
  - Drapes
  - A 10-mL syringe
  - Sponges to clean the insertion area with antiseptic
  - A 1-in. #22 gauge needle
  - A ⅝-in. #25 gauge needle for the local anesthetic
  - A scalpel
  - Forceps
  - Two rubber-tipped clamps for each tube inserted
  - Several 4 × 4 gauze squares
  - Split drain gauzes
  - A chest tube with a trocar
  - Suture materials (eg, 2-0 silk with a needle)
- A pleural drainage system with sterile drainage tubing and connectors
- A Y-connector, if two tubes will be inserted
- Sterile gloves for the physician and the nurse
- A vial of local anesthetic (eg, 1% lidocaine)
- Alcohol sponges to clean the top of the vial

- Antiseptic (eg, povidone-iodine)
- Tape (nonallergenic is preferable)
- Sterile petrolatum gauze (optional) to place around the chest tube

Set up the drainage system so it is ready for use.

For tube removal:

- Clean gloves to remove the dressing
- Sterile gloves to remove the tube
- A sterile suture removal set, with forceps and suture scissors
- Sterile petrolatum gauze
- Several 4 × 4 gauze squares
- Air-occlusive tape, 2 or 3 in. wide (nonallergenic is preferred)
- Scissors to cut the tape
- An absorbent linen-saver pad
- A moistureproof bag
- Sterile swabs or applicators in sterile containers to obtain a specimen (optional)

INTERVENTION

1. Obtain baseline assessment data.

Chest Tube Insertion

2. Assist the client to a lateral position with the area to receive the tube facing upward. Determine from the physician whether to have the bed in the supine position or semi-Fowler's position.

   Rationale A supine position is generally preferred for tube insertion into the second or third intercostal space, a semi-Fowler's position for the sixth to eighth intercostal spaces.

3. Open the chest tube tray and the sterile gloves on the overbed table. Pour antiseptic solution onto the sponges. Be sure to maintain sterile technique.

4. Wipe the stopper of the anesthetic vial with an alcohol sponge. After the physician dons the gloves and cleans the insertion area with anti-

septic solution, invert the vial and hold it for the physician to withdraw the anesthetic.

5. Support and monitor the client as required, while the physician anesthetizes the area, makes a small incision, inserts the tube, either clamps the tube or immediately connects it to the drainage system, and then sutures the tube to the skin.

6. Optional: Don sterile gloves. Wrap a piece of sterile petrolatum gauze around the chest tube. Place drain gauzes around the insertion site (one from the top and one from the bottom). Place several 4 × 4 gauze squares over these.

   Rationale The gauze makes an airtight seal at the insertion site.

7. Remove your gloves, if donned, and tape the dressings, covering them completely.

8. Tape the chest tube to the client's skin away from the insertion site.

   Rationale Taping prevents accidental dislocation of the tube.

9. Tape the connections of the chest tube to the drainage tube and to the drainage system.

   Rationale Taping prevents inadvertent separation.

10. Coil the drainage tubing, and secure it to the bed linen, ensuring enough slack for the person to turn and move.

    Rationale This prevents kinking of the tubing and impairment of the drainage system.

11. When all drainage connections are completed, ask the client to
    a. Take a deep breath and hold it for a few seconds.
    b. Slowly exhale.

       Rationale These actions facilitate drainage from the pleural space and lung reexpansion.

12. Assess the client's vital signs every 15 minutes for the first hour following tube insertion and then as ordered, eg, every hour for 2 hours, then every 4 hours or as often as health indicates.

13. Auscultate the lungs at least every 4 hours for breath sounds and the adequacy of ventilation in the affected lung.

14. Place rubber-tipped chest tube clamps at the bedside.

    Rationale These are used to clamp the chest tube and prevent pneumothorax if the tube becomes disconnected from the drainage system or the system breaks or cracks.

15. Assess the client regularly for signs of pneumothorax and subcutaneous emphysema. Go to step 30.

Chest Tube Removal

16. Administer an analgesic, if ordered, 30 minutes before the tube is removed.

17. Ensure that the chest tube is securely clamped.

    Rationale Clamping prevents air from entering the pleural space.

18. Assist the client to a semi-Fowler's position or to a lateral position on the unaffected side.

19. Put the absorbent pad under the client beneath the chest tube.

    Rationale The pad protects the bed linen from drainage and provides a place for the chest tube after removal.

20. Open the sterile packages, and prepare a sterile field.

21. Wearing sterile gloves, place the sterile petrolatum gauze on a 4 × 4 gauze square.

    Rationale This will quickly provide an airtight dressing over the insertion site after the tube is removed.

22. Remove the soiled dressings, being careful not to dislodge the tube. Remove the underlying gauzes, which may contain drainage. Discard soiled dressings in the moisture-resistant bag.

23. The physician will
    a. Don sterile gloves.
    b. Hold the chest tube with forceps.
    c. Cut the suture holding the tube in place.
    d. Instruct the client to either inhale or exhale fully and hold the breath while removing the tube.

       Rationale This prevents air from being sucked into the pleural space during tube removal.
    e. Place the prepared petrolatum gauze dressing over the insertion site immediately after tube removal.

24. While the physician is removing the tube, remove gloves and prepare three 15-cm (6-in.) strips of air-occlusive tape.

25. After the gauze dressing is applied, completely cover it with the air-occlusive tape.

    Rationale This makes the dressing as airtight as possible.

26. If a specimen is required for culture and sensitivity, use a swab to obtain drainage from inside the chest tube, while the physician holds the tube.

27. Monitor the vital signs, and assess the quality of the respirations as health indicates, eg, every 15 minutes for the first hour following tube removal and then less often.

28. Auscultate the client's lungs every hour for the first 4 hours to assess breath sounds and the adequacy of ventilation in the affected lung.

29. Assess the client regularly for signs of pneumothorax, subcutaneous emphysema, and infection.

30. Document the date and time of chest tube insertion or removal and the name of the physician. For insertion, document the insertion site, drainage system used, presence of bubbling, vital signs, breath sounds by auscultation, and any other assessment findings. For removal, document the amount, color, and consistency of drainage, vital signs, and the specimen obtained for culture, if taken.

Sample Recording

Date	Time	Notes
12/6/89	2200	Sudden sharp pain in L chest, diaphoretic, pale, and dyspneic.———————
	2300	BP 100/70, TPR 98.6, 105, 24. Diminished breath sounds in L lung and absence of chest movement. Two chest tubes inserted by Dr. Jung in L 2nd and 8th ICS. Connected by Y-connector and attached to Pleur-evac. Drainage system functioning.———————
	2305	BP 110/70, TPR 98.6, 100, 20. Breath sounds present in L lung.—————— ———————Karen P. Smith, RN

Sample Recording

Date	Time	Notes
12/12/89	1000	Chest tubes removed by Dr. Jung. 100 mL clear pink drainage. BP 120/70, TPR 98.6, 76, 16. Specimen of chest tube drainage taken for culture and sensitivity and sent to lab.—Susan March, NS

PROCEDURE 42–10 Monitoring a Client with Chest Drainage

Policies and procedures vary considerably from agency to agency in regard to chest drainage interventions. Certain interventions, such as milking a chest tube to maintain patency, may be prohibited. The nurse must therefore review agency policies before intervening.

EQUIPMENT

- Two rubber-tipped Kelly clamps
- A sterile petrolatum gauze
- A sterile drainage system
- Antiseptic swabs
- Sterile 4 × 4 gauzes
- Air-occlusive tape
- A mechanical chest tubing stripper, if ordered
- Specimen supplies, if needed:
  - A povidone-iodine swab
  - A sterile #18 or #20 gauge needle
  - A 3- or 5-mL syringe
  - A needle protector
  - A label for the syringe
  - A laboratory requisition

INTERVENTION

1. Obtain baseline assessment data.

Safety precautions

2. Keep two 15- to 18-cm (6- to 7-in.) rubber-tipped Kelly clamps within reach at the bedside, to clamp the chest tube in an emergency, eg, if leakage occurs in the tubing.

3. Keep one sterile petrolatum gauze within reach at the bedside to use with an air-occlusive material if the chest tube becomes dislodged.

4. Keep an extra drainage system unit available in the client's room. In most agencies the physician is responsible for changing the drainage system except in emergency situations, such as malfunction or breakage. In these situations:
   a. Clamp the chest tubes (see step 6).

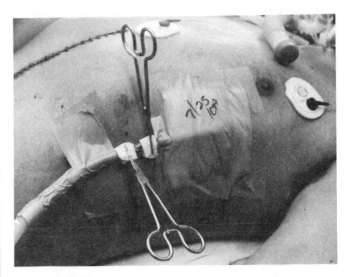

Figure 42–18

   b. Reestablish a water-sealed drainage system.
   c. Remove the clamps, and notify the physician.

5. Keep the drainage system below chest level and upright at all times, unless the chest tubes are clamped.

   Rationale Keeping the unit below chest level prevents backflow of fluid from the drainage chamber into the pleural space. Keeping the unit upright maintains the glass tube below the water level, forming the water seal.

6. If the chest tube becomes disconnected from the drainage system:
   a. Have the client exhale fully.
   b. Clamp the chest tube close to the insertion site with two rubber-tipped clamps placed in opposite directions. See Figure 42–18.
   c. Quickly clean the ends of the tubing with an antiseptic, reconnect them, and tape them securely.
   d. Unclamp the tube as soon as possible.
   e. Assess the client closely for respiratory distress.

   Rationale Clamping the tube prevents external air from entering the pleural space. Two clamps ensure complete closure of the tube. Having the client exhale and clamping the tube for no longer than necessary prevents an air or fluid buildup in the pleural space, which can cause further lung collapse.

7. If the chest tube becomes dislodged from the insertion site:

   a. Remove the dressing, and immediately apply pressure with the petrolatum gauze, your hand, or a towel.

   b. Cover the site with sterile 4 × 4 gauze squares.

   c. Tape the dressings with air-occlusive tape.

   d. Notify the physician immediately.

   e. Assess the client for respiratory distress every 15 minutes or as health indicates.

8. Do not empty a drainage bottle unless there is an order to do so. Commercial systems cannot be emptied.

9. If the drainage system is accidentally tipped over:

   a. Immediately return it to the upright position.

   b. Ask the client to take several deep breaths.

   Rationale Deep breaths help force air out of the pleural cavity that might have entered when the water seal was not intact.

   c. Notify the nurse in charge and the physician.

   d. Assess the client for respiratory distress.

Monitoring and Maintaining the Drainage System

10. Check that all connections are secured with tape to ensure that the system is airtight.

11. Milk or strip the chest tubing *as ordered and only in accordance with agency protocol.* Too vigorous milking can create excessive negative pressure that can harm the pleural membranes and/or surrounding tissues. Always verify the physician's orders before milking the tube; milking of only short segments of the tube may be specified (eg, 10–20 cm or 4–8 in.). To milk a chest tube, use a mechanical stripper (see Figure 42–19), or follow these steps:

    a. Lubricate about 10–20 cm (4–8 in.) of the drainage tubing with lubricating gel, soap, or hand lotion, or hold an alcohol sponge between your fingers and the tube.

    Rationale Lubrication reduces friction and facilitates the milking process.

    b. With one hand, securely stabilize and pinch the tube at the insertion site.

    c. Compress the tube with the thumb and forefinger of your other hand and milk it by sliding them down the tube, moving away from the insertion site.

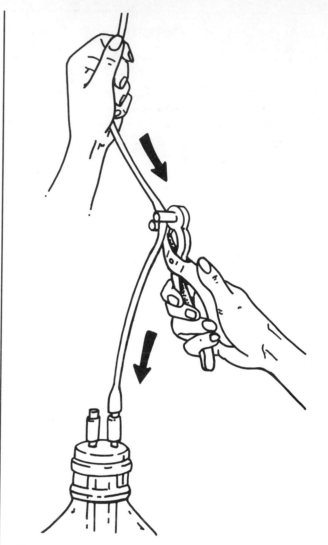

Figure 42–19

Rationale Milking the tubing dislodges obstructions such as blood clots. Milking from the insertion site downward prevents movement of the obstructive material into the pleural space.

    d. If the entire tube is to be milked, reposition your hands farther along the tubing, and repeat steps a–c in progressive overlapping steps, until you reach the end of the tubing.

12. Inspect the drainage in the collection container at least every 30 minutes during the first 2 hours after chest tube insertion and every 2 hours thereafter. Every 8 hours mark the time, date, and drainage level on a piece of adhesive tape affixed to the container, or mark it directly on a disposable container (see Figure 42–20). Note any sud-

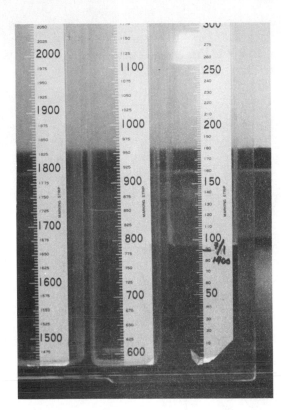

Figure 42–20

den change in the amount or color of the drainage. If drainage exceeds 100 mL/hour or if a color change indicates hemorrhage, notify the physician immediately.

13. In gravity drainage systems, check for fluctuation (tidaling) of the fluid level in the water-seal glass tube of a bottle system or the water-seal chamber of a commercial system as the client breathes. Normally, fluctuations of 5–10 cm (2–4 in.) occur until the lung has reexpanded. In suction drainage systems, the fluid line remains constant.

    Rationale Fluctuations reflect the pressure changes in the pleural space during inhalation and exhalation. The fluid level rises when the client inhales and falls when the client exhales. The absence of fluctuations may indicate tubing obstruction from a kink, dependent loop, blood clot, or outside pressure (eg, because the client is lying on the tubing), or may indicate that full lung reexpansion has occurred.

14. To check for fluctuation in suction systems, temporarily disconnect the system. Then observe the fluctuation.

15. Check for intermittent bubbling in the water of the water-seal bottle or chamber.

    Rationale Intermittent bubbling normally occurs when the system removes air from the pleural space, especially when the client takes a deep breath or coughs. Absence of bubbling indicates that the pleural space has healed and is sealed. Continuous bubbling or a sudden change from an established pattern can indicate a break in the system and should be reported immediately.

16. Check for gentle bubbling in the suction-control bottle or chamber.

    Rationale Gentle bubbling indicates proper suction pressure.

17. Inspect the air vent in the system periodically to make sure it is not occluded. A vent must be present to allow air to escape.

    Rationale Obstruction of the air vent causes an increased pressure in the system that could result in pneumothorax.

18. Inspect the drainage tubing for kinks or loops dangling below the entry level of the drainage system.

Detecting Air Leaks

Continuous bubbling in the water-seal collection chamber normally occurs for only a few minutes after a chest tube is attached to drainage, since fluid and air initially rush out from the intrapleural space under high pressure. Continuous bubbling that persists indicates an air leak.

19. To determine the source of an air leak follow the next steps sequentially:

    a. Check the tubing connection sites. Tighten and retape any connection that seems loose.

       Rationale The tubing connection sites are the most likely places for leaks to occur. Bubbling will stop if these are the source of the leak.

    b. If bubbling continues, clamp the chest tube near the insertion site and see if the bubbling stops while the client takes several deep breaths. Chest tube clamping must be done only for a few seconds at a time.

       Rationale Clamping the chest tube near the insertion site will help determine whether the leak is proximal or distal to the clamp. Clamping for long periods can aggravate an existing pneumothorax or lead to a recurrent pneumothorax.

    c. If bubbling stops, follow step 20. The source of the air leak is above the clamp, ie, between the clamp and the client. It may be either at the insertion site or inside the client.

   d. If bubbling continues, follow step 21. The source of the air leak is below the clamp, ie, in the drainage system below the clamp.

20. To determine whether the air leak is at the insertion site or inside the client:

   a. Unclamp the tube and palpate gently around the insertion site. If the bubbling stops, the leak is at the insertion site. To remedy this situation, apply a petrolatum gauze and a 4 × 4 gauze around the insertion site and secure these dressings with adhesive tape.

   b. If the leak is not at the insertion site, it is inside the client and may indicate a dislodged tube or a new pneumothorax, a new disruption of the pleural space. In this instance leave the tube unclamped, notify the physician, and monitor the client for signs of respiratory distress.

21. To locate an air leak below the chest tube clamp:

   a. Move the clamp a few inches farther down and keep moving it downward a few inches at a time. Each time the clamp is moved, check the water-seal collection chamber for bubbling. The bubbling will stop as soon as the clamp is placed between the air leak and the water-seal drainage.

   b. Seal the leak when you locate it by applying tape to that portion of the drainage tube.

   c. If bubbling continues after the entire length of the tube is clamped, the air leak is in the drainage device. To remedy this situation the drainage system must be replaced and the physician notified.

Client Care

22. Encourage deep-breathing and coughing exercises every 2 hours. Have the client sit upright to perform the exercises, and splint the tube insertion site with a pillow or with a hand to minimize discomfort.

   Rationale Deep breathing and coughing help to remove accumulations from the pleural space, facilitate drainage, and help the lung to reexpand.

23. While the client takes deep breaths, palpate the chest for thoracic expansion. Place your hands together at the base of the sternum so that your thumbs meet. As the client inhales, your thumbs should separate at least 2.5–5 cm (1–2 in.). Note whether chest expansion is symmetric.

24. Reposition the client every 2 hours. When the client is lying on the affected side, place rolled towels beside the tubing.

   Rationale Frequent position changes promote drainage, prevent complications, and provide comfort. Rolled towels prevent occlusion of the chest tube by the client's weight.

25. Assist the client with range-of-motion exercises of the affected shoulder three times per day to maintain joint mobility.

26. When transporting and ambulating the client:

   a. Attach rubber-tipped forceps to the client's gown for emergency use.

   b. Keep the water-seal unit below chest level and upright.

   c. If it is necessary to clamp the tube, remove the clamp as soon as possible.

   d. Disconnect the drainage system from the suction apparatus before moving the client, and make sure the air vent is open.

Taking a Specimen of Chest Drainage

27. Specimens of chest drainage may be taken from a disposable chest drainage system, since these systems are equipped with self-sealing ports. If a specimen is required:

   a. Use a povidone-iodine swab to wipe the self-sealing diaphragm on the back of the drainage collection chamber. Allow it to dry.

   b. Attach a sterile #18 or #20 gauge needle to a 3- or 5-mL syringe, and insert the needle into the diaphragm.

   c. Aspirate the specimen, attach the needle protector, label the syringe, and send it to the laboratory with the appropriate requisition form.

| PROCEDURE 42–11 | **Clearing an Obstructed Airway** |

There are several possible causes of airway obstruction and, as a result, several different ways of clearing an obstructed airway. Causes include

- Aspirated food, mucus plug, or foreign bodies, such as partial dentures or small toys. Food is the most common cause of choking, particularly meat that has been ineffectively chewed.

- Unconsciousness or seizures, which cause the tongue to fall back and block the airway.

- Severe trauma to the nose, mouth, or neck that produces blood clots that obstruct the airway, especially in unconscious victims.

- Acute edema of the trachea, from smoke inhalation, facial and neck burns, or anaphylaxis. In these instances, a tracheostomy is often indicated.

Foreign bodies may cause either partial or complete airway obstruction.

When an airway is partially obstructed, the victim may either have good air exchange or poor air exchange. If sufficient air is obtained, even though there is frequent wheezing between coughs, do not interfere with the victim's attempts to expel the foreign object. If the partial obstruction remains, call the emergency medical service (EMS). Partial obstructions with inadequate air exchange are dealt with in the same manner as complete obstructions.

The victim with complete airway obstruction is unable to speak, breathe, or cough and may clutch at the neck. The *Heimlich maneuver* (subdiaphragmatic abdominal thrusts) is recommended to relieve the obstruction for persons over 1 year of age. By elevating the diaphragm, this maneuver forces air from the lungs to create an artificial cough to expel the obstruction. It may be necessary to perform this maneuver 6–10 times to clear the airway. The Heimlich maneuver can be performed when the victim is conscious and standing or sitting, or when the victim is unconscious and lying flat. For infants under 1 year of age, a combination of back blows and chest thrusts is recommended. The Heimlich maneuver can cause intraabdominal injury in this age group.

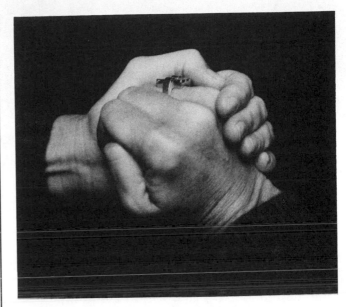

Figure 42–21

INTERVENTION

Heimlich Maneuver to a Standing or Sitting Victim

To perform the Heimlich maneuver to a conscious person who is standing or sitting:

1. Stand behind the person, and wrap your arms around the person's waist.

2. Make a fist with one hand, tuck the thumb inside the fist, and place the flexed thumb against the person's epigastrium, ie, below the xiphoid process. A protruding thumb could inflict injury.

3. With the other hand, grasp the fist (see Figure 42–21), and press it into the person's abdomen with a firm, quick upward thrust (see Figure 42–22). Avoid tightening the arms around the rib cage, and thrust in the direction of the chin. Deliver one quick thrust.

4. Deliver successive thrusts as separate and complete movements.

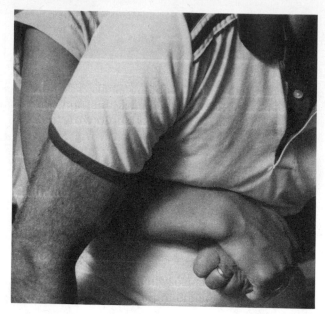

Figure 42–22

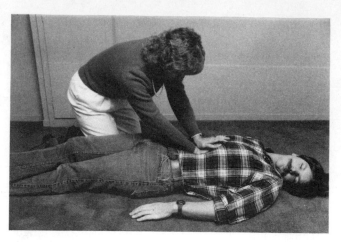

Figure 42–23

Heimlich Maneuver to a Victim Lying on the Ground

To implement the Heimlich maneuver to an unconscious person who is lying on the ground:

5. Place the person supine and kneel preferably astride or to the side of the person's thighs.

6. Place the heel of one hand slightly above the person's navel and well below the tip of the xiphoid process, ie, in the epigastric area.

7. Place the other hand directly on top of the first. Make sure the shoulders are over the person's abdomen and the elbows are straight.

8. Press the heel of the first hand into the abdomen with a quick upward thrust. See Figure 42–23. Be sure to direct the thrust in the midline of the abdomen and not to the left or to the right. The weight of your shoulders and trunk supplies power for the thrust.

Chest Thrusts to Standing or Sitting Victims

Chest thrusts are to be administered only to women in advanced stages of pregnancy and markedly obese persons who cannot receive the Heimlich maneuver. To administer chest thrusts:

9. Stand behind the person with your arms under the person's armpits and encircling the person's chest.

10. Place the thumb side of the fist on the *middle* of the breast bone, not on the xiphoid process.

11. Grab the fist with the other hand and deliver a quick backward thrust.

12. Repeat thrusts until the obstruction is relieved.

Chest Thrust to a Victim Lying Flat

Chest thrusts to unconscious persons lying on the ground are administered only to women in advanced stages of pregnancy or markedly obese persons. To administer this maneuver:

13. Position the person supine and kneel close to the side of the person's trunk.

14. Position the hands as for cardiac compression with the heel of the hand on the lower half of the sternum. (See Procedure 42–13, steps 1–4.)

15. Administer downward thrusts, each one slow and distinct.

Back Blows and Chest Thrusts for Infants

To administer a combination of back blows and chest thrusts to infants:

16. Straddle the infant over your forearm with his or her head lower than the trunk.

17. Support the infant's head by firmly holding the jaw in the hand.

18. Rest your forearm on your thigh.

19. With the heel of the free hand, deliver four sharp blows to the back over the spine between the scapulae. See Figure 42–24.

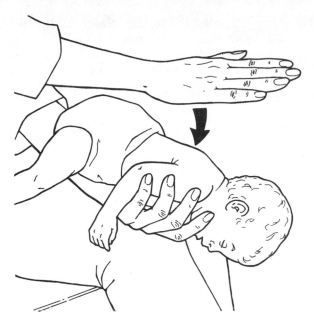

Figure 42–24

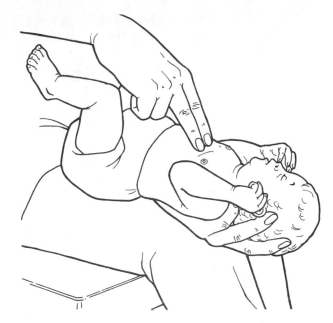

Figure 42–25

20. Turn the infant as a unit to the supine position:
    a. Place the free hand on the infant's back.
    b. While continuing to support the jaw, neck, and chest with the other hand, turn and place the infant on the thigh with the baby's head lower than the trunk.

21. Using two or three fingers, administer four chest thrusts over the sternum in the same location as external chest compression for cardiac massage, ie, one finger width below the nipple line. See Figure 42–25.

22. Assess whether the infant has effective air exchange. If not, repeat the series of back blows and abdominal or chest thrusts until there is effective air exchange.

Variation: Placement over the Lap

An alternate method to administer back blows and chest thrusts involves placing the infant over your lap:

23. Lay the infant face down over your thighs with the baby's head lower than the trunk and firmly supported.

24. Administer four back blows, turn the infant as a unit to the supine position, and administer four chest thrusts as described earlier.

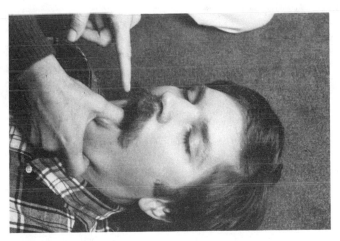

Figure 42–26

Finger Sweep

If foreign material is visible in the mouth it must be expediently removed. The finger sweep maneuver should be used only on unconscious persons and with extreme caution in infants and children since the foreign material can be pushed back into the airway, causing increased obstruction. To digitally remove visible foreign material from the mouth:

25. Don disposable gloves.

26. Open the person's mouth by grasping the tongue and lower jaw between the thumb and fingers, and lifting the jaw upward. See Figure 42–26.

    Rationale This pulls the tongue away from the back of the throat.

27. To remove solid material insert the index finger of your free hand along the inside of the person's cheek and deep into the throat. With your finger hooked, use a sweeping motion to try to dislodge and lift out the foreign object. If these measures fail, try more abdominal thrusts and back blows.

28. After removing the foreign object, clear out liquid material, such as mucus, blood, or emesis, with a scooping motion, using two fingers wrapped with a tissue or piece of cloth.

29. After the digital maneuver, assess air exchange.

PROCEDURE 42–12 **Administering Oral Resuscitation**

Oral resuscitation is achieved in four ways: by mouth-to-mouth, mouth-to-nose, and mouth-to-mouth-and-nose resuscitation, or by the use of a hand-compressible breathing bag (eg, the Ambu bag).

Mouth-to-mouth resuscitation depends on the large amount of air that a normal person can inhale and therefore breathe into the victim's lungs. Although the oxygen content of expired air is slightly reduced, it is sufficient for revival.

A current problem facing resuscitators relates to the AIDS epidemic. The Occupational Safety and Health Administration (OSHA) is recommending that health care workers avoid direct contact with the skin, mucous membranes, blood, blood products, excretions, secretions, and tissue of possible AIDS victims. Health care personnel should use breathing-bag-and-mask ventilation rather than mouth-to-mouth resuscitation and wear gloves. Check local policies and recommendations.

EQUIPMENT

- A hand-compressible breathing bag and mask, if available or recommended. See Figure 42–27.

INTERVENTION

1. Obtain baseline assessment data.

2. Ensure that the client's mouth and throat are cleared of any obstructive material. See "Finger Sweep" in Procedure 42–11.

   Rationale A clear airway prior to resuscitation permits air to move freely in and out of the respiratory passages.

3. If the person is lying on one side or face down, turn the client onto the back, and kneel beside the head.

Opening the Airway

4. Open the airway by using the head-tilt, chin-lift maneuver or the jaw thrust maneuver. See steps 5–6. A modified jaw thrust is used for victims with suspected neck injury. See step 7.

   Rationale In unconscious persons the tongue lacks sufficient muscle tone, falls to the back of the throat, and obstructs the pharynx. Because the tongue is attached to the lower jaw, moving

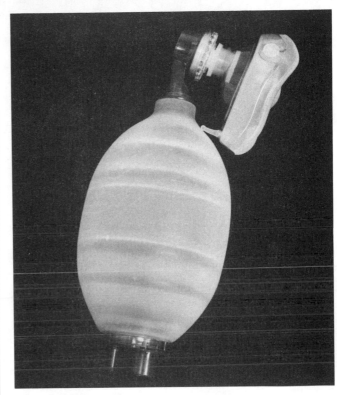

Figure 42–27
An Ambu bag with face mask.

the lower jaw forward and tilting the head backward lifts the tongue away from the pharynx and opens the airway. See Figure 42–28.

5. *Head-tilt, chin-lift maneuver:*

   a. Place one hand palm downward on the forehead.

   b. Place the fingers of the other hand under the bony part of the lower jaw near the chin. The teeth should then be almost closed. The mouth should *not* be closed completely.

   c. Simultaneously press down on the forehead with one hand, and lift the person's chin upward with the other. See Figure 42–29. Avoid pressing the fingers deeply into the soft tissues under the chin since too much pressure can obstruct the airway.

   d. Open the person's mouth by pressing the lower lip downward with the thumb after tilting the head.

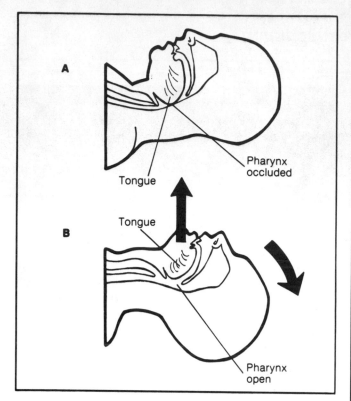

Figure 42-28

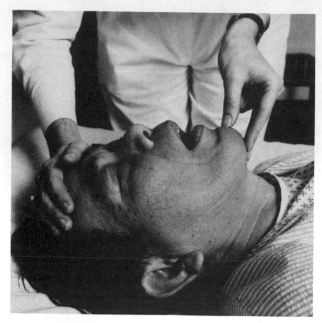

Figure 42-29

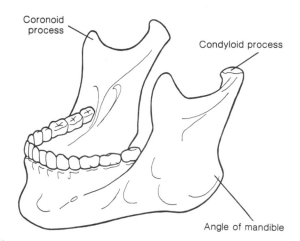

Figure 42-30

e. Remove dentures if they cannot be maintained in place. However, dentures that can be maintained in place make a mouth-to-mouth seal easier should rescue breathing be required. Go to step 8.

   or

6. *Jaw-thrust maneuver:*
   a. Kneel at the top of the victim's head.
   b. Grasp the angle of the mandible directly below the earlobe between your thumb and forefinger on each side of the person's head. See Figure 42-30.
   c. While tilting the head backward, lift the lower jaw until it juts forward and is higher than the upper jaw. See Figure 42-31.
   d. Rest your elbows on the surface on which the person is lying.
   e. Retract the lower lip with the thumbs prior to giving artificial respiration.

7. If the victim is suspected of having a spinal neck injury, do not hyperextend the neck. Instead, *use the modified jaw thrust for a person with a spinal injury:*
   a. Perform steps 6a and 6b.

   b. Do not tilt the head backward while lifting the lower jaw forward.
   c. Support the head carefully without hyperextending it or moving it from side to side.

8. Check the person's breathing. See the assessment guide (Breathing) for this chapter.

9. If no breathing is evident, rescue breathing must be initiated. Try to blow air into the person's lungs by using one of the methods in steps 10-13.

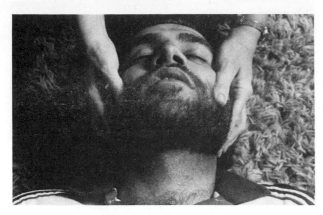

Figure 42–31

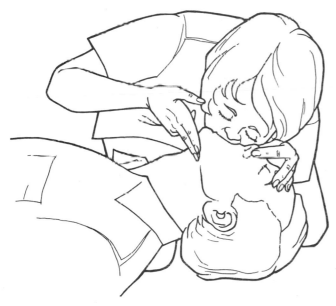

Figure 42–32

Rescue Breathing

10. *Mouth-to-mouth method:*
    a. Maintain the open airway by using the head-tilt, chin-lift maneuver.
    b. Pinch the person's nostrils with the index finger and thumb of the hand on the person's forehead.
       Rationale Pinching closes the nostrils and prevents resuscitation air from escaping through them.
    c. Take a deep breath, and place the mouth, opened widely, around the victim's mouth. Ensure an airtight seal. See Figure 42–32.

   d. Exhale two full breaths ($1-1\frac{1}{2}$ seconds per breath). Pause and take a breath after the first ventilation.
      Rationale The 1- to $1\frac{1}{2}$-second time span closely matches the victim's inspiratory time, allows adequate time to provide good chest expansion, and decreases the possibility of gastric distention. Excessive air volumes and rapid inspiratory flow rates can cause pharyngeal pressures that are great enough to open the esophagus, thus allowing air to enter the stomach.
   e. Ensure adequate ventilation by observing the person's chest rise and fall and by assessing the person's breathing as outlined in the assessment guide. Adequate ventilation volumes for most adults are about 800 mL and do not need to exceed 1200 mL.
   f. If the initial ventilation attempt is unsuccessful, reposition the person's head and repeat the rescue breathing as above. If the victim still cannot be ventilated, proceed to clear the airway of any foreign bodies. See Procedure 42–11.

   or

11. *Mouth-to-nose method:* This method can be used when there is an injury to the mouth or jaw or when the client is *edentulous*, making it difficult to achieve a tight seal over the mouth.
    a. Maintain the head tilt and chin lift.
    b. Close the person's mouth by pressing the palm of your hand against the person's chin. The thumb of the same hand may be used to hold the bottom lip closed.
    c. Take a deep breath, and seal your lips around the person's nose. Ensure a tight seal by making contact with the cheeks around the nose.
    d. Deliver two full breaths of $1-1\frac{1}{2}$ seconds each and pause to inhale before delivering the second breath.
    e. Remove your mouth from the nose and allow the victim to exhale passively. It may be necessary to separate the victim's lips or to open the mouth for exhaling, since the nasal passages may be obstructed during exhalation. Go to step 14.

   or

12. *Mouth-to-mouth-and-nose method:* This method is used for infants and children.
    a. Place your mouth tightly over the infant's nose and mouth.

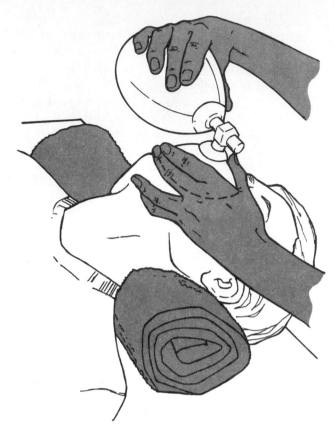

Figure 42-33

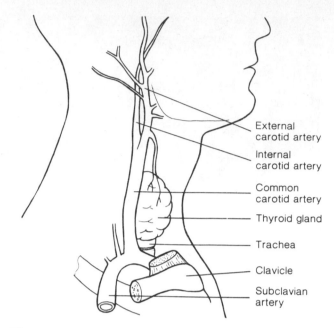

External
carotid artery

Internal
carotid artery

Common
carotid artery

Thyroid gland

Trachea

Clavicle

Subclavian
artery

Figure 42-34

b. Deliver two slow breaths of $1-1\frac{1}{2}$ seconds each and pause to inhale before delivering the second breath. An appropriate ventilation volume is that which makes the chest rise and fall.

or

13. *Hand-compressible breathing bag method:* Many agencies provide rubberized breathing bags (eg, the Ambu bag) attached to face masks for respiratory resuscitation. The bags are compressed by hand to deliver air into the mask and rapidly self-inflate after compression. Exhaled air is released through an exhaust valve to prevent its entry back into the bag. Two significant advantages of the breathing bag are that supplemental oxygen can be attached to it and the nurse avoids direct contact with the person's mouth or nose. To use a breathing bag:

a. Stand at the person's head.

b. Use one hand to secure the mask at the top and bottom and to hold the person's jaw forward. Use the other hand to squeeze and release the bag. See Figure 42-33.

c. Compress the bag until sufficient elevation of the person's chest is observed. Then release the bag.

14. Determine whether the client's breathing is restored.

15. Determine the person's carotid pulse by palpating the common carotid artery. See Figure 42-34. (Use the brachial pulse for an infant.) Adequate time is needed for this pulse check (about 5-10 seconds), since the victim's pulse may be very weak and rapid, irregular, or slow.

Rationale Since the carotid arteries carry about one-fourth of the total normal blood flow, bringing it to the brain, a pulse can often be palpated there when more peripheral pulses, such as the radial, are imperceptible. Gentle pressure avoids compressing the artery. The carotid pulse is used since the femoral pulse is difficult to locate on a fully clothed person. In hospitals health practitioners may prefer to use the femoral pulse.

16. If the carotid pulse is palpable, but breathing is not restored, repeat step 9, and inflate the lungs at the rate of 12 breaths per minute (1 breath every 5 seconds). Blow forcibly enough to make the person's chest rise. If chest expansion fails to occur, ensure that the head is hyperextended and the jaw lifted upward, or check again for the presence of obstructive material, fluid, or vomitus. For infants and small children, provide 1 breath every 3 seconds, using only sufficient force to cause the chest to rise.

17. After each inflation, move your mouth away from the person's mouth by turning your head toward the person's chest.

    Rationale This movement allows the air to escape when the person exhales. It also gives the nurse time to inhale and to watch for chest expansion.

18. Reassess the carotid pulse after every 12 inflations (after 1 minute). For an infant, reassess the brachial pulse after every 20 inflations (after 1 minute). If you cannot locate the pulse, the person's heart has stopped, and cardiac compression also needs to be provided. See Procedure 42–13. Accurate assessment of the person's pulse is essential since performing external chest compressions on victims who have a pulse can lead to serious medical complications.

PROCEDURE 42–13 **Administering External Cardiopulmonary Resuscitation to an Adult**

The external chest compression procedure consists of sequential, rhythmic applications of pressure over the lower half of the sternum. These compressions provide circulation to the lungs, heart, brain, and other organs through increased intrathoracic pressure and/or direct compression of the heart. The heart is squeezed between the sternum and the vertebrae lying posteriorly. Cardiac compression is ineffective unless there is simultaneous artificial respiration to oxygenate the bloodstream.

External cardiac compression should never be practiced on a person with a functioning heart, because it could interfere with the normal cardiac contractions.

The ABCs of cardiopulmonary resuscitation are

A. Clear the *airways*.
B. Initiate artificial *breathing* (oral resuscitation).
C. Initiate cardiac compression, or artificial *circulation*.

This sequence is recommended because spontaneous breathing may occur after any one action, such as after the airway is opened or after a few artificial respirations are provided.

Each of the ABCs of CPR begins with an assessment phase:

A. *Airways:* Determine the person's air exchange and responsiveness.
B. *Breathing:* Determine the person's breathlessness.
C. *Circulation:* Determine the person's pulselessness.

Performing each assessment step ensures that the person will not be subjected to any intrusive procedure (eg, positioning, opening the airway, rescue breathing, external cardiac compression) until the need for it is determined.

EQUIPMENT

- A cardiac board if available. The headboard or footboard of a hospital bed often can be removed and used.

- An Ambu bag if available.

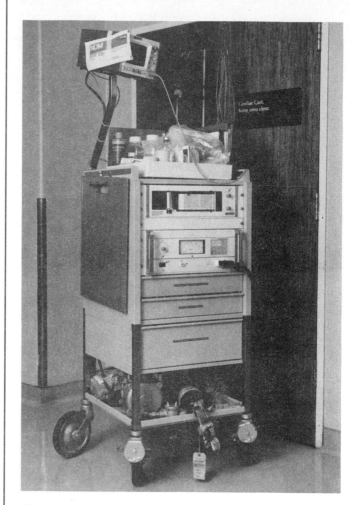

Figure 42–35
A crash (emergency) cart.

- A crash (emergency) cart if available. See Figure 42–35. The cart generally contains a defibrillator, cardiac monitor, and the following supplies:
  - Airway equipment.
  - Prepackaged medications.
  - Intravenous supplies.
  - Blood tubes, needles, syringes, and blood gas kits.
  - Laboratory requisitions.
  - Suction equipment.

INTERVENTION

Hand Placement

Proper hand placement is essential for effective cardiac compression. Position the hands as follows:

1. With the hand nearest the victim's legs, use your middle and index fingers to locate the lower margin of the rib cage.

2. Move the fingers up the rib cage to the notch where the ribs meet the sternum. See Figure 42–36.

3. Place the heel of the other hand (nearest the victim's head) along the lower half of the victim's sternum, close to the index finger that is next to the middle finger in the costal-sternal notch.

   Rationale Proper positioning of the hands during cardiac compression prevents injury to underlying organs and the ribs. See Figure 42–37. Compression directly over the xiphoid process can lacerate the person's liver.

4. Then place the first hand on top of the second hand so that both hands are parallel. The fingers may be extended or interlaced.

   Rationale Compression occurs only on the sternum through the heels of the hands.

Compression Technique

The method of cardiac compression recommended by the American Heart Association is achieved as follows:

5. Lock your elbows into position, straighten your arms, and position your shoulders directly over your hands. See Figure 42–38.

6. For each compression, thrust *straight down* on the sternum. For an adult of normal size, depress the sternum 3.8–5.0 cm (1.5–2 in.).

   Rationale The muscle force of both arms is needed for adequate cardiac compression of an adult. The weight of your shoulders and trunk supplies power for compression. Extension of the elbows ensures an adequate and even force throughout compression. The pressure compresses the heart between the sternum and the vertebral column and squeezes blood out of the chambers of the heart.

7. Completely release the compression pressure. However, do *not* lift your hands from the chest or change their position.

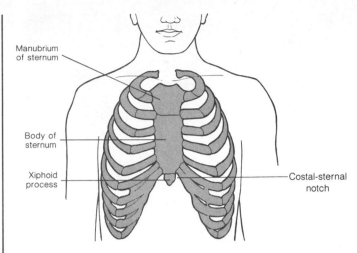

Manubrium of sternum

Body of sternum

Xiphoid process

Costal-sternal notch

Figure 42–36

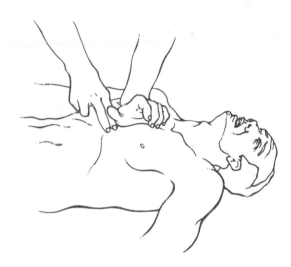

Figure 42–37

Rationale Releasing the pressure allows the sternum to return to its normal position and allows the heart chambers to fill with blood. Leaving the hands on the chest prevents taking a malposition between compressions and possibly injuring the person.

8. Provide external cardiac compressions at the rate of 80–100 per minute. Maintain the rhythm by counting "One and, two and," etc.

   Rationale The specified compression rate and rhythm simulate normal heart contractions.

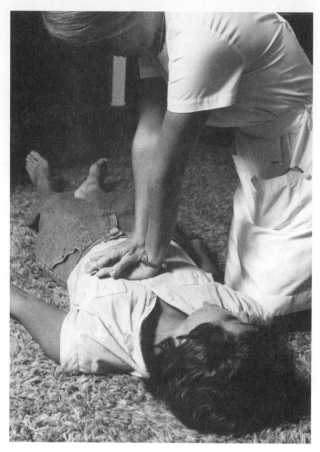

Figure 42–38

CPR Performed by One Rescuer

9. Assess responsiveness.

10. Call for help and have another person call for EMS. In many communities the emergency telephone number is 911. The American Heart Association recommends that the person who calls the local EMS be able to impart all of the following information:

    a. Location of the emergency
    b. Telephone number from which the call is being made
    c. What happened
    d. Number of people needing assistance
    e. Condition of the victim(s)
    f. What aid is being given
    g. Any other information that is requested

    If no help comes and the rescuer is alone, CPR should be performed for 1 minute and then help summoned.

11. Position the client on the back on a flat, firm surface. Place a cardiac board, if available, under the back of a person in bed. If necessary, place the person on the floor. Elevate the lower extremities (optional). If the person must be turned, turn as a unit. Firmly support the head and neck so that the head does not roll, twist, or tilt backward or forward.

    Rationale Blood flow to the brain will be inadequate during CPR if the victim's head is positioned higher than the thorax. A hard surface facilitates compression of the heart between the sternum and the hard surface. Elevating the lower extremities may promote venous return and augment circulation during external cardiac compressions. The person is turned as a unit to prevent further injury (if present) to the neck or spine.

12. Kneel beside the person's chest. If the person is in bed, you may have to kneel on the bed.

Airway

13. Clear the airway if you suspect airway obstruction from food or some other foreign object. See Procedure 42–11 for detailed steps.

14. Open the airway with the head-tilt, chin-lift maneuver or if neck injury is suspected, use the modified jaw thrust.

    Rationale This prevents the tongue from occluding the airway.

Breathing

15. Assess breathing: *Look* for chest movement; *listen* for exhalation; and *feel* for air flow against the cheek.

16. Ventilate the person, if breathing is not restored. See Procedure 42–12 for detailed steps.

17. Deliver two full breaths into the person's mouth. See Procedure 42–12. Between the breaths, remove your mouth, turn your head to the side, and pause to take a breath.

    Rationale Turning away allows the nurse to take a fresh breath, allows the person to exhale, and enables the nurse to observe the person's chest rise and fall.

18. If unable to give two breaths, then reposition the client's head and attempt to ventilate again.

19. If still unsuccessful, remove foreign bodies from the victim's airway. See digital removal of material from the mouth in Procedure 42–11.

Circulation

20. Assess the carotid or femoral pulse for 5 seconds.

21. If pulse is present:
    a. Continue rescue breathing at 12 times per minute while monitoring the pulse.
    b. Call for EMS.

22. If pulse is absent:
    a. Call for EMS.
    b. Begin external chest compression.
    c. Perform chest compression: 15 external chest compressions at the rate of 80–100 per minute. Count, "One and, two and, three and . . ." up to 15.
    d. Open the airway and give two rescue breaths.
    e. Repeat 15 chest compressions.
    f. Perform four complete cycles of 15 compressions and two ventilations.

23. Assess the client's carotid pulse after four sets of 15 compressions, each followed by two lung inflations. If there is no pulse, continue with CPR and check for return of pulse every few minutes. Do not interrupt CPR for more than 7 seconds.

CPR Performed by Two Rescuers

When help arrives, one rescuer can provide external cardiac compression, and the other can provide pulmonary resuscitation, inflating the lungs once after every five compressions, a 5:1 ratio. The second rescuer follows these initial steps:

24. Tell the first rescuer, "Stop CPR after two ventilations."

25. Check the carotid or femoral pulse for 5 seconds.

26. If no pulse is felt, state, "No pulse."

27. The second rescuer then
    a. Gives two breaths.
    b. Provides compression.
    c. Sets the pace, counting aloud, "One and, two and, three and, four and, five and, ventilate."

28. The first rescuer:
    a. Provides one ventilation after every five chest compressions.
    b. Observes each breath for effectiveness.
    c. Assesses the carotid pulse frequently between breaths to assess the effectiveness of cardiac compression.
    d. Observes for abdominal (gastric) distention, which can result from overinflation of the lungs. If distention occurs, the rescuer reduces the force of the ventilations, but ensures sufficient ventilation to elevate the ribs.
    e. Assesses the person's pupils every 5 minutes (optional). Pupil changes are not the best indicator of restored circulation, however.

29. When the person compressing the chest becomes fatigued, positions should be changed. To initiate a change in positions, the person compressing states, "Change one and, two and, three and, four and, five and"; moves to the person's head; and counts the pulse for 5 seconds. CPR should never be interrupted for more than 7 seconds.

30. The person ventilating gives the breath and moves into position to provide compression.

31. If there is no pulse, the original person compressing states, "No pulse–start compression," gives one full breath, and CPR is again initiated.

When Relieved from CPR

32. Stand by to assist. Often a person is needed to take notes, document the actions taken, and record the drugs given by the cardiac arrest team.

33. Provide support to the victim's support persons and others who may have witnessed the cardiac arrest. This is often a frightening experience for others because it is so sudden and so serious.

34. Document the time CPR began, the time a physician arrived, the drugs and techniques employed, the time CPR was terminated, and all nursing assessments.

Terminating CPR

A rescuer terminates CPR only when one of the following events occurs:

- Another person takes over.
- The victim's heartbeat and breathing are reestablished.
- Adjunctive life-support measures are initiated.
- A physician states that the individual is dead and that CPR is to be discontinued.
- The rescuer becomes exhausted, and there is no one to take over.

Sample Recording

Date	Time	Notes
12/5/89	0315	CPR initiated by Rose R. Sach RN and Earl L. Nunn LPN. Client placed on cardiac board. CPR at 5 compressions to 1 inflation. Code 99 called.————————————Wayne P. Newman, RN
	0320	No carotid pulse. Pupils dilated. Skin pale, moist.————
	0322	Dr. R. Sanduriz and crash team arrived.
	0340	Femoral pulse 68, regular, adequate volume.————
	0345	Respirations started 10/min. CPR terminated. Carotid pulse 72. Color pink. Reacts to verbal stimuli. BP 100/40. Pupils react and equal.————Wayne P. Newman, RN
	0350	Dr. Sanduriz phoned Dr. Saunders.————
	0355	BP 110/55, P 76. Color pink. Condition stable. ————Wayne P. Newman, RN

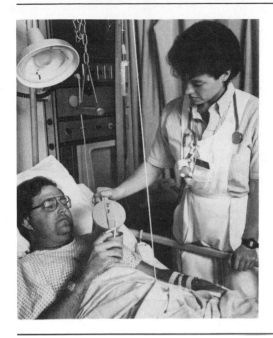

CHAPTER 43

FLUIDS AND ELECTROLYTES

☐ The following procedures appear in *Introduction to Nursing:*

Procedure 43–1
Monitoring Fluid Intake and Output

Procedure 43–2
Using an Infusion Pump or Controller

Procedure 43–3
Changing an Intravenous Container and Tubing

■ New procedures:

Procedure 43–4
Setting Up an Intravenous Infusion

Procedure 43–5
Discontinuing an Intravenous Infusion.

PROCEDURE 43–4 **Setting Up an Intravenous Infusion**

Setting up or preparing an intravenous infusion primarily involves readying the client and assembling the equipment. Agency practices vary about personnel allowed to perform venipunctures.

EQUIPMENT

- The container(s) of sterile intravenous solution. IV solutions are supplied in bottles and plastic bags. See Figure 43–1.
  - Select the size ordered if possible. Intravenous solutions are supplied in 150-mL, 250-mL, 500-mL, and 1000-mL sizes, but some agencies, for economic reasons, stock only 1000-mL containers. If a 1000-mL solution container *must* be used, when 750 mL are ordered, for example, remove 250 mL before starting the IV. Too often the incorrect amount can be instilled.
  - Some solution bottles have a tube inside the bottle that serves as an air vent so that, as the solution runs out of the bottle, it is replaced with air. See Figure 43–2. Containers without air vents require a vent on the administration set. See Figure 43–3. Air vents usually have filters to remove any contamination from the air that enters the container.

- An administration set, consisting of an insertion spike, a drip chamber, a roller or screw clamp, tubing, and a protective cap over the needle adapter. See Figure 43–4. The insertion spike is kept sterile and inserted into the solution container when the IV is set up and ready to start. The drip chamber permits a predictable amount of fluid to be delivered to the client. A commonly used drip chamber is the macrodrip, which provides 10, 15, or 20 drops per mL of solution. This information will be on the package. There are also microdrip or minidrip sets, which provide 60 drops per mL of solution. The roller or screw clamp is used to control the rate of flow of the solution by compressing the lumen of the tubing. The protective cap over the needle adapter maintains the sterility of the end of the tubing so that it can be attached to a sterile needle inserted in the client's vein.

- IV poles (rods) for hanging the solution container. Some poles are attached to hospital beds. Others stand on the floor or hang from the ceiling. There are floor models with casters that can be pushed along when a client is up and walking. The height

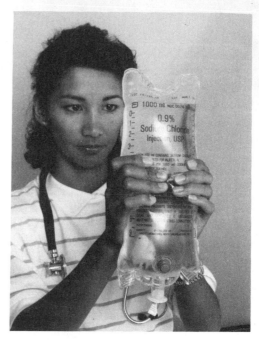

Figure 43–1
A plastic intravenous fluid container.

of most poles is adjustable. The higher the solution container is suspended, the greater the force of the solution as it enters the client and the faster the rate of flow.

- An intravenous needle or catheter. These are usually packaged separately. Butterfly, or wing-tipped needles, with wings attached to the shaft, are commonly used. See Figure 43–5. They vary in length from 1.5–3 cm (½–1 ¼ in.) and from #25–17 gauge in diameter. (The larger the gauge number, the smaller the diameter of the shaft.) Needles of #20–22 gauge and short lengths are commonly used for adults. Some practitioners prefer to use a needle bevel that is short, to minimize injury to the tissues and discomfort on insertion. A catheter or angiocatheter is a plastic tube that is inserted into the client's vein. Some catheters fit over a needle during insertion, while others fit inside a needle. See Figure 43–6. An angiocatheter has a metal stylet (needle), which is used to pierce the skin and vein and is then withdrawn, leaving the catheter in place.

- An arm board if needed to help immobilize the client's arm. Arm boards are made of plastic, metal, or wood. They are usually padded with a towel, for

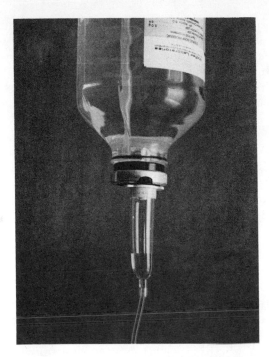

Figure 43–2
An intravenous container with an indwelling vent. Note that the administration set does not have a vent.

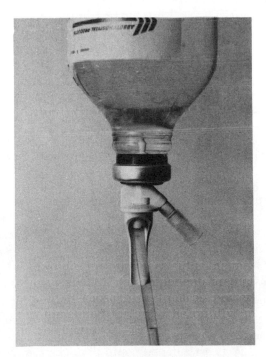

Figure 43–3
An intravenous container without an indwelling vent. Note the vent on the tubing just below the container.

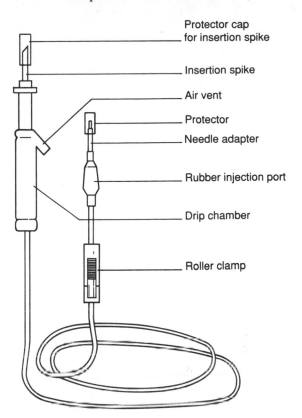

Protector cap for insertion spike

Insertion spike

Air vent

Protector

Needle adapter

Rubber injection port

Drip chamber

Roller clamp

Figure 43–4
An intravenous administration set, consisting of an insertion spike with a protector cap, an air vent (optional), a drip (drop) chamber, plastic tubing with a roller control clamp, rubber injection port, and a needle adapter covered by a protective cap.

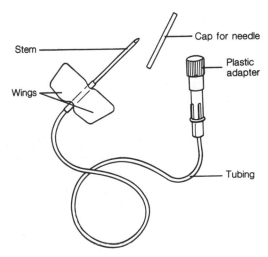

Stem

Wings

Cap for needle

Plastic adapter

Tubing

Figure 43–5
An intravenous butterfly (wing-tipped) needle.

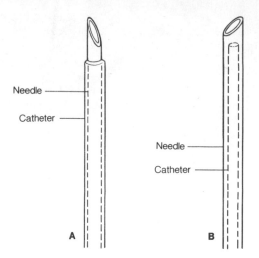

Figure 43–6
A: An over-the-needle catheter. After insertion in the vein, the needle is removed, and the plastic catheter remains. **B:** An inside-the-needle catheter (intracatheter). The plastic catheter is threaded through the needle after the venipuncture.

comfort. Tape or wrapping is required to secure the board to the client's arm.

- An intravenous tray containing all the supplies required to start an IV. It should include sterile swabs, antiseptic solution, plastic or paper tape, and a tourniquet.

- Sterile 2 × 2 gauze squares and/or transparent tape to place over the insertion site.

- A local anesthetic (eg, 1% lidocaine without epinephrine) and a small syringe with a #27 gauge needle, if this is to be used before the venipuncture.

Additional equipment is required for variations from the standard infusion. Secondary sets are required when more than one solution is running at the same time.

- In a tandem setup, a second container is attached to the line of the first container at the lower, secondary port. See Figure 43–7, A. It permits medications to be administered intermittently or simultaneously with the first solution.

- In the piggyback alignment, a second set connects the second container to the tubing of the first at the upper port. This setup is used solely for intermittent drug administration. See Figure 43–7, B. Various manufacturers describe these sets differently, so check the manufacturer's labeling and directions carefully.

- Another variation is a volume-control set, which is used if the volume of fluid administered is to be carefully controlled. The set is attached below the solution container, and the drip chamber is placed below it. See Figure 43–8. Volume-control sets are frequently used in pediatric settings, where the volume administered is critical.

Agencies have different policies about when to take the equipment to the bedside prior to starting an intravenous infusion. Normally, it is not taken to the bedside in advance if it will produce anxiety in the client.

INTERVENTION

1. Determine from the order the type of solution, the amount to be administered, and the rate of flow of the infusion. Most agencies use abbreviations to describe commonly used solutions, eg, DW (distilled water), NS (normal saline), D5W (5% dextrose in water), D5NS (5% dextrose in normal saline).

2. Determine from the order if any special equipment is required, eg, a microdrip set is usually required if the fluid is to be administered at a rate of 50–75 mL/hr or less, for accurate regulation.

3. Determine the type of needle or catheter to be used.

4. Determine what equipment is contained in an intravenous set. Some agencies have special trays for use by personnel who start infusions. These are normally kept in a central place and taken to the bedside when the infusion is to be started.

5. Explain the procedure to the client. A venipuncture can cause discomfort for a few seconds, but there should be no discomfort while the solution is flowing. People often want to know how long the process will last. The order may specify the length of time of the infusion, eg, 3000 mL over 24 hours.

6. Provide any scheduled care before establishing the IV, to minimize movement of the affected limb during the procedure, since moving the limb after the IV is established could dislodge the needle.

7. Make sure that the client's gown can be removed over the IV apparatus if necessary. Some agencies provide special gowns that open over the shoulder and down the sleeve for easy removal.

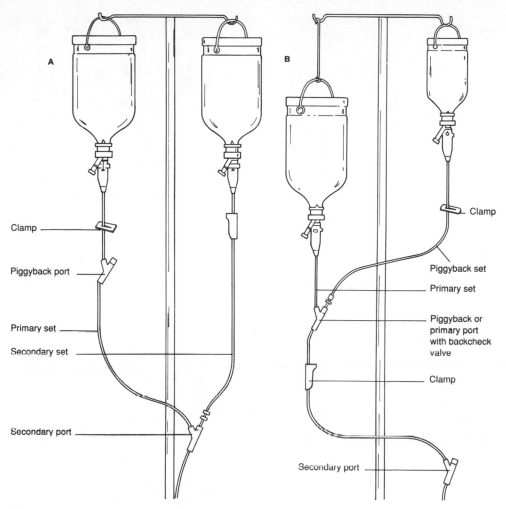

Figure 43–7
A: A tandem intravenous alignment. The secondary set connects to the secondary (lower) port of the primary set. **B:** A piggyback intravenous alignment. The secondary set connects to the primary (upper) port of the primary set.

8. Determine that the solution is sterile and in proper condition, ie, clear. Check the expiration date on the label. There should be no particulate matter in the solution and the vacuum seal should be intact. Also, nurses should not write on the bag because the ink may seep into the solution. Examine the other packages to confirm their sterility. Inspect and squeeze a plastic solution bag for any leaks or hairline cracks. Return any unsatisfactory container to the central supply or distributing department, indicating the reason for the return.

Rationale Cloudiness, evidence that the container has been opened previously, or leaks indicate possible contamination.

9. Open the administration set, maintaining the sterility of the ends of the tubing. The ends of the tubing may be covered with plastic caps, which are left in place until the IV is started.

10. Slide the tubing clamp along the tubing until it is just below the drip chamber.

11. Close the clamp.

12. If using an intravenous bottle with a rubber stopper, remove the metal disc while maintaining the sterility of the stopper. If the stopper becomes contaminated while you are removing the metal disc, swab it with disinfectant. Remove the cap from the tubing, and insert the spike firmly

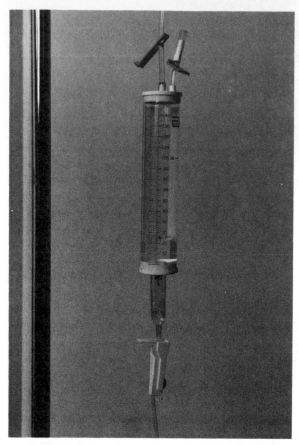

Figure 43–8
A volume-control set above the drip chamber of an
intravenous infusion.

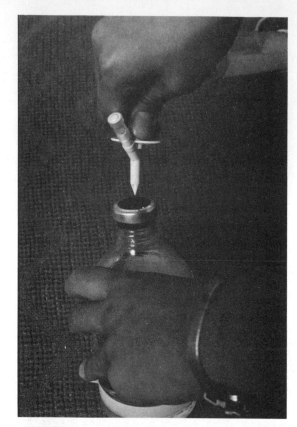

Figure 43–9

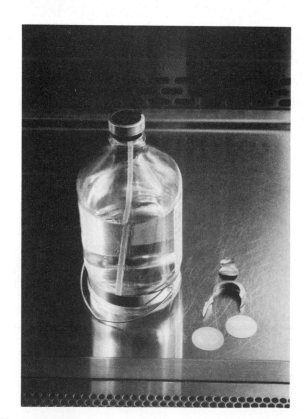

Figure 43–10

through the rubber stopper into the port, maintaining sterile technique. See Figure 43–9.
or
If using a bottle with an indwelling vent, remove
the metal disc and the rubber diaphragm, keeping the stopper sterile. Listen for a hissing sound
as the air rushes into the bottle. If there is no
hissing sound, discard the container because it
was probably not sealed. Insert the spike into the
larger hole (the one without the vent). See Figure
43–10.
or
For spiking a plastic bag, read the manufacturer's
directions. Some bags are hung on the pole before
spiking.

13. Hang the solution container on the pole, usually
about 1 m (3 ft) above the client's head.

Rationale This height is needed to enable gravity to overcome venous pressure and facilitate
flow of the solution into the vein.

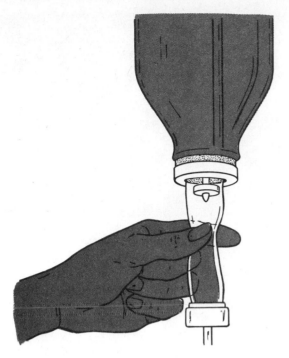

Figure 43-11

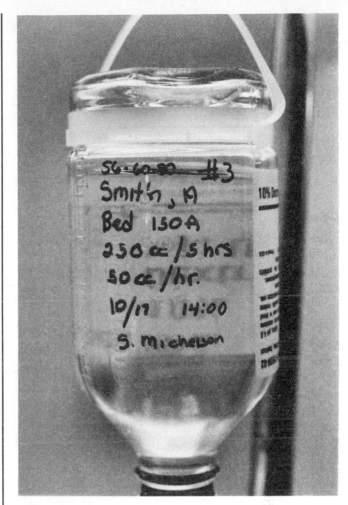

56-60-80   #3
Smith, A
Bed 150A
250 cc/5 hrs
50 cc/hr.
10/17   14:00
S. Michelson

Figure 43-12

14. If using a flexible drip chamber, squeeze it gently until it is half full of solution. See Figure 43-11.
    or
    If the drip chamber is firm, it will usually fill automatically.

    Rationale The drip chamber is partly filled with solution to prevent air from moving down the tubing. Also, the lovol of solution must be below the dropper of the drip chamber for effective monitoring and functioning of the system.

15. To prime the tubing, remove the protective cap, and hold the tubing over a cup or basin. Maintain the sterility of the end of the tubing and the cap. Release the clamp and let the fluid run through the tubing until all bubbles are removed. Tap the tubing with your fingers to help the bubbles move.

    Rationale The tubing is primed to prevent the introduction of air into the client, because air bubbles can act as emboli in the bloodstream.

16. Reclamp the tubing.

17. Replace the tubing cap, maintaining sterile technique.

18. Label the solution container, applying the label upside down on the container. Include the following information: the client's name, identification number, room, and/or bed number; any medication and dosage; the drip rate; the date, the time the container is being started; the con-

tainer number; and the name of the person starting it. See Figure 43-12. Labeling may be done when the IV is started.

    Rationale The label is applied upside down so it can be read easily when the container is hanging up. The IV bottles are numbered consecutively.

19. Apply a timing label on the solution container. See Figure 43-13. The timing label may be applied at the time the IV is started. Follow agency practice.

20. Label the IV tubing with the date and time of attachment. See Figure 43-14. This labeling may also be done at the time the IV is started.

    Rationale The tubing is labeled to ensure that it is changed every 48 hours or as agency policy dictates.

21. Assess the client's reaction to the setting up of the IV. If the client expresses anxiety and fear, assist the person to deal with the emotions, and record your assessments and interventions.

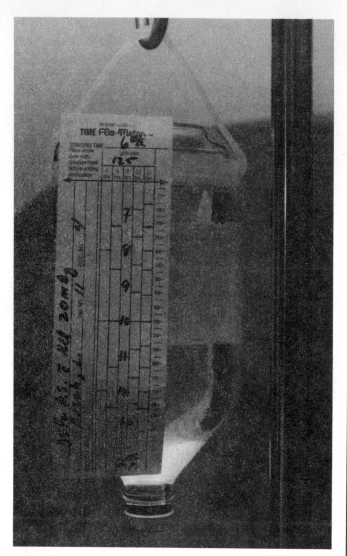

Figure 43–13

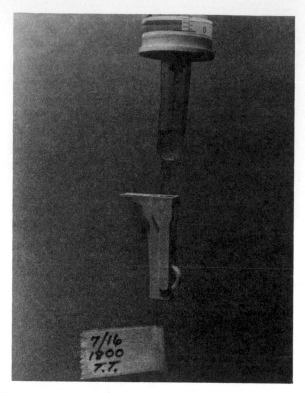

Figure 43–14

22. Notify the nurse in charge when the intravenous infusion has been set up.

23. Assist with starting the IV as needed.

PROCEDURE 43–5 **Discontinuing an Intravenous Infusion**

Discontinuing an infusion is not uncomfortable; in fact, it is usually a relief for the client and takes only a couple of minutes. IVs are usually discontinued for one of three reasons:

- The client's oral fluid intake and hydration status are satisfactory so that no further intravenous solutions are ordered.
- There is a problem with the infusion that cannot be fixed. Consult with the nurse in charge before discontinuing an IV because of such a difficulty.
- The medications administered by the intravenous route (eg, antibiotics) are no longer required.

EQUIPMENT

- A small sterile dressing and tape to cover the site temporarily
- Dry or antiseptic-soaked swabs, according to agency practice
- Gloves to protect the nurse from contamination by the client's body secretions

INTERVENTION

1. Clamp the infusion tubing.

   Rationale Clamping the tubing will prevent the fluid from flowing out of the needle onto the client or bed.

2. Loosen the tape at the venipuncture site while holding the needle firmly and applying countertraction to the skin.

   Rationale Movement of the needle can injure the vein and cause discomfort to the client. Countertraction prevents pulling the skin and causing discomfort.

3. Don gloves and hold a swab above the venipuncture site.

4. Withdraw the needle or catheter by pulling it out along the line of the vein.

   Rationale Pulling out in line with the vein avoids injury to the vein.

5. Immediately apply firm pressure to the site, using the swab, for 2–3 minutes.

   Rationale Pressure helps stop the bleeding and prevents hematoma formation.

6. Hold the client's arm or leg above the body if any bleeding persists.

   Rationale Raising the limb decreases blood flow to the area.

7. Check the needle or catheter to make sure it is intact. Report a broken needle or catheter to the nurse in charge immediately. If the broken piece can be palpated, apply a tourniquet above the insertion site.

   Rationale If a piece of needle or tubing remains in the client's vein it could move centrally (toward the heart or lungs) and cause serious problems. Application of a tourniquet decreases the possibility of the piece moving until a physician is notified.

8. Apply the sterile dressing.

   Rationale The dressing continues the pressure and covers the open area in the skin, preventing infection.

9. Assess the client's response to the IV in terms of the appearance of the venipuncture site; the pulse, respirations, color, edema, sputum, cough, and urine output; and how the person feels physically and psychologically.

10. Discard the IV solution container, if infusions are being discontinued, and discard the used supplies appropriately.

11. Record the amount of fluid infused on the intake and output record and on the chart, according to agency practice. Include the container number, type of solution used, time of discontinuing the infusion, and the client's response.

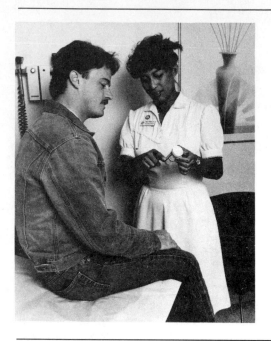

MEDICATIONS

PROCEDURE 44–9 **Mixing Medications in One Syringe**

Frequently, clients need more than one drug injected at the same time. To spare the client the experience of being injected twice, two drugs (if compatible) are often mixed together in one syringe and given as one injection. For instance, two types of insulin may be combined in this manner. Or, injectable preoperative medications, such as morphine or meperidine (Demerol) with atropine or scopolamine, may be combined. Drugs may be mixed from two vials, from two ampules, or from one vial and one ampule. Drugs may also be mixed in intravenous solutions. When uncertain about drug compatibilities, the nurse should consult a pharmacist before mixing the drugs.

Insulins should only be combined as directed by the physician or pharmacist. In some cases the simultaneous injection of two insulin preparations in one syringe provides essentially the same effect that is obtained from the injection of the same quantities of the preparation into different sites. However, the insulins must be of the same species and of equal purity to be combined. For example, Novolin-Toronto Human should only be mixed with Novolin-Lente, Novolin-NPH, or Novolin-Ultralente. The order of mixing and brand or model of syringe should also be specified. As a general rule, short-acting insulins should be drawn into the syringe first.

EQUIPMENT

- The client's medication cards, computer printout, or chart. Confirm that they correspond with the physician's order.

- Two vials of medication, or one vial and one ampule, or one vial and one cartridge. Note that insulin is prepared in units rather than milligrams or grains. It is available in 100 units/mL of solution. It is essential when preparing insulin that the appropriate syringe be used. In the hospital, insulin may be stored in the refrigerator to prevent deterioration.

- Sterile hypodermic or insulin syringe and needle. If insulin is being given, use a small-gauge hypodermic needle (#26 gauge).

- Additional sterile subcutaneous or intramuscular needle (optional).

- Sterile antiseptic-soaked swabs.

INTERVENTION

Mixing Medications from Two Vials

1. Inspect the appearance of the medication for clarity. Some medications are normally cloudy.

   Rationale Preparations that have changed in appearance should be discarded.

2. If using insulin, thoroughly mix the solution in each vial prior to administration. Rotate the vials between the palms of the hands and invert the vials.

   Rationale Mixing ensures an adequate concentration and thus an accurate dose. Shaking insulin vials can make the medication frothy, making precise measurement difficult.

3. Clean the tops of the vials with disinfectant swabs.

4. Inject a volume of air equal to the volume of medication to be withdrawn into vial A or into the vial of longer-acting insulin, eg, NPH insulin. See Figure 44–1, step 1.

   Rationale The same needle is used to inject air into and withdraw medication from the second vial. It must not be contaminated with the medication in vial A.

5. Withdraw the needle from vial A, and inject the prescribed amount of air into vial B or into the vial of shorter-acting insulin (eg, regular or crystalline zinc insulin). See Figure 44–1, step 2.

6. Withdraw the required amount of medication from vial B. See Figure 44–1, step 3.

7. Using a newly attached sterile needle, withdraw the required amount of medication from vial A. See Figure 44–1, step 4. If using a syringe with a fused needle, withdraw the medication from Vial A. The syringe now contains a mixture of medications from vials A and B.

   Rationale With this method, neither vial is contaminated by microorganisms or by medication from the other vial.

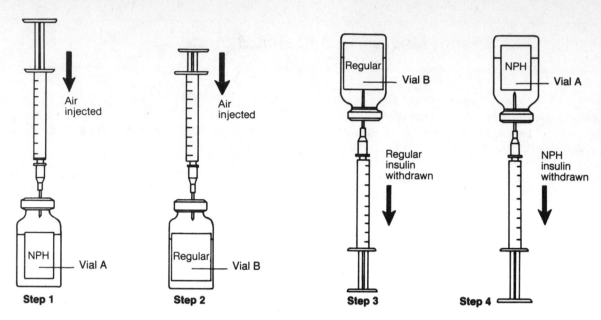

Figure 44–1

Mixing Medications from One Vial and One Ampule

8. First prepare and withdraw the medication from the vial.

Rationale   Ampules do not require the addition of air prior to withdrawal of the drug.

9. Then withdraw the required amount of medication from the ampule.

PROCEDURE 44–10 **Administering an Intradermal Injection**

An intradermal (intracutaneous) injection is the administration of a drug into the dermal layer of the skin just beneath the epidermis. Usually, only a small amount of liquid is used, eg, 0.1 mL. This method of administration is frequently indicated for allergy and tuberculin tests and for vaccinations. Common sites for intradermal injections are the inner lower arm, the upper chest, and the back beneath the scapulae. See Figure 44–2.

EQUIPMENT

- The medication card or computer printout.

- A vial or ampule of the correct sterile medication.

- A sterile syringe and needle. A $\frac{1}{2}$-in., #25 gauge needle is generally used.

- Acetone and 2 × 2 sterile gauze square (optional).

- Alcohol swab. A colorless antiseptic that will not hinder the reading of the test is used.

- A dry sterile gauze pad.

INTERVENTION

1. Check the physician's orders carefully for the medication, dosage, and route.

2. Determine the agency's practices about how to prepare the injection site. Some agencies defat the skin with acetone before disinfecting the area with alcohol.

3. Prepare the medication. See Procedure 44–2 in *Introduction to Nursing.*

4. Explain that the medication will produce a small bleb like a blister. The client will feel a slight prick as the needle enters the skin. Some medications are absorbed slowly through the capillaries into the general circulation, and the bleb gradually disappears. Other drugs remain in the area and interact with the body tissues to produce redness and induration (hardening), which will need to be interpreted at a particular time, eg, in 24 or 48 hours. This reaction will also gradually disappear.

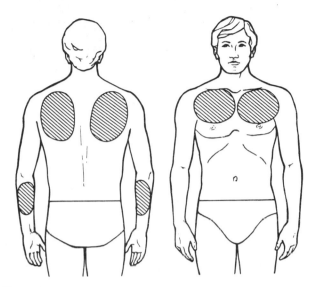

Figure 44–2
Sites of the body commonly used for intradermal injections

5. If the client feels faint, assist the person to either a sitting or lying position as a precaution.

6. Inspect the skin at the injection site for abrasions, localized inflammation, redness, tenderness, hardness, swelling, scarring, itching, or burning. Avoid using such sites.

7. Defat the skin with acetone if agency policy dictates, using a gauze square or swab moistened with acetone. Start at the center and widen the circle outward.

8. Using the same method, clean the site with an antiseptic swab. Allow the area to dry thoroughly.

   Rationale Recommendations differ about the necessity of cleaning the skin prior to injections. See Procedure 44–3, step 4, in *Introduction to Nursing.*

9. Remove the needle cap while waiting for the antiseptic to dry.

10. Expel any air bubbles from the syringe. Small bubbles that adhere to the plunger are of no consequence, since a small amount of air will not harm the tissues.

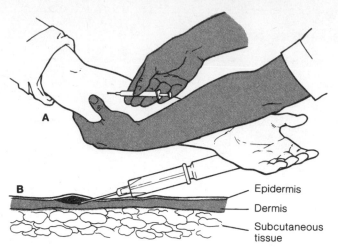

Epidermis
Dermis
Subcutaneous tissue

Figure 44–3

11. Grasp the syringe in your dominant hand, holding it between thumb and four fingers, with your palm upward. Hold the needle at a 15° angle to the skin surface, with the bevel of the needle up.

12. With the nondominant hand, pull the skin at the site until it is taut, and thrust the tip of the needle firmly through the epidermis into the dermis. See Figure 44–3, *A*. Do not aspirate.

13. Inject the medication carefully so that it produces a small bleb on the skin. See Figure 44-3, *B*.

14. Withdraw the needle quickly while providing countertraction on the skin, and wipe the injection site gently with a dry sterile gauze pad. Do not massage the area.

    Rationale A dry sterile gauze is used since alcohol interferes with some diagnostic skin tests. Massage can disperse the medication into the tissue or out through the needle insertion site.

15. Assess the client at the time the drug is expected to act.

16. Document the medication given, including the time, dosage, route, site, and nursing assessments.

PROCEDURE 44–11   **Administering an IV Medication by Using Additive Sets**

Because IV medications enter the client's bloodstream directly, they are appropriate when a rapid effect is required (eg, in a life-threatening situation such as a cardiac arrest). The IV route is also appropriate when medications are too irritating to tissues to be given by other routes, eg, levarterenol bitartrate (Levophed) for acute hypotension. When an IV line is already established, this route is desirable because it avoids the discomfort of other parenteral routes.

There are, however, potential hazards in giving IV medications: infection and rapid, severe reactions to the medication. To prevent infection, sterile technique is used during all aspects of IV medication administration. To safeguard the client against severe reactions, the nurse must administer the drug slowly, following the manufacturer's recommendations. The client must be assessed closely during the administration, and the medication is discontinued immediately if an untoward reaction occurs.

Additional fluid containers and sets are sometimes attached to a primary infusion set to administer IV medications. They may be used intermittently to administer IV drugs that cannot be mixed with the primary solution for reason of incompatibility. Or, they may be used to maintain peak levels of a medication in the client's bloodstream and at the same time maintain a constant total infusion rate by simultaneous infusion of the primary line.

There are two means of attaching additional containers: the piggyback set and the secondary set. The piggyback set (see Figure 44–4, *B*) consists of a small IV bottle (minibottle) and a short tubing line that is connected to the upper Y-port (the piggyback port) of the primary line. Either a macrodrip or a microdrip system may be used, but usually a macrodrip system is used. The term *piggyback* refers to the positioning of the additive bottle, which is higher than the primary infusion bottle. Manufacturers provide an extension hook to position the primary bottle below the piggyback bottle. The piggyback set is used for intermittent IV drug administration. Antibiotics are most commonly administered by the piggyback infusion.

The secondary set (see Figure 44–4, *A*) uses a second microdrip or macrodrip bottle of any size and a long tubing line that is attached to the lower Y-port (secondary port) of the primary line. The primary and secondary bottles are positioned at the same height. This system is used to administer IV drugs intermittently or continuously with the primary IV solution.

EQUIPMENT

- The appropriate additive set.
- The physician's order, medication card, or computer printout.
- The correct sterile medication.
- A sterile syringe and needle. Generally, a #20 gauge, 1-in. needle is used because longer needles can puncture the tubing and cause leakage of IV fluid.
- A medication label.
- An antiseptic swab.
- Adhesive tape.

INTERVENTION

1. Check the physician's orders carefully for the medication, dosage, and route.

2. Ascertain whether the medication is compatible with the primary infusion and with any other medications that are to be added.

3. Determine how the additive set is to be attached and, if a secondary set is used, whether it is to run simultaneously with the primary infusion or if the primary infusion is to be clamped off at the time.

4. Prepare the medication according to Procedure 44–2 in *Introduction to Nursing*.

5. Insert the medication into the additional container. See Procedure 44–5 in *Introduction to Nursing*.

Using a Piggyback Set

6. Spike the piggyback administration set into the top of the piggyback bottle.

7. Attach the 1-in. needle to IV tubing, prime the tubing, and close the clamp.

8. Label the tubing with the date and time it is established.

9. Clean the piggyback port on the primary IV line with an antiseptic swab.

10. Verify that the medication to be administered is compatible with the primary IV solution. If the

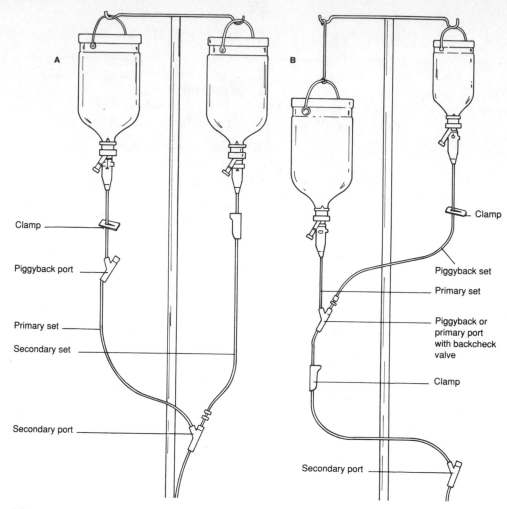

Figure 44–4
A: A tandem intravenous alignment. The secondary set connects to the secondary (lower) port of the primary set. **B:** A piggyback intravenous alignment. The secondary set connects to the primary (upper) port of the primary set.

medication is not compatible with the primary infusion, flush the primary line with a sterile saline solution before attaching the secondary set. To flush the line, wipe the port with an antiseptic swab, clamp the primary line, and, using a sterile needle and syringe, instill a few milliliters of sterile saline through the port to wash any primary infusion fluid out of the infusion tubing.

11. If the medication is compatible, insert the piggyback needle into the piggyback port on the primary line and secure it with adhesive tape. Some agencies recommend that a needle guard be taped alongside the needle to support the needle placement and keep the needle guard handy for use when discontinuing the secondary attachment.

12. Using the extension hook, reposition the primary container so that it is lower than the piggyback container.

13. Open the clamp on the piggyback line, and regulate it in accordance with the recommended rate for that medication. When a piggyback set is used, a backcheck valve in the port automatically stops the flow of the primary infusion so that only the additive set infuses. See Figure 44–5. After the piggyback solution has infused and the level of the solution is below the level of the primary infusion drip chamber, the backcheck valve is released, and the primary infusion automatically starts running.

14. Go to step 22.

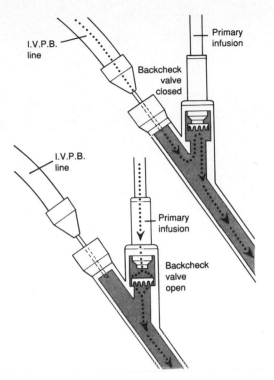

I.V.P.B. line

Primary infusion

Backcheck valve closed

I.V.P.B. line

Primary infusion

Backcheck valve open

Figure 44–5

Using a Secondary Set

15. Spike the secondary administration set into the top of the secondary bottle.

16. Attach the 1-in. needle to the IV tubing, prime the tubing, and close the clamp.

17. Label this tubing with the date and time it is attached.

18. Clean the secondary port on the primary IV line with an antiseptic swab.

19. Verify that the medication to be administered is compatible with the primary IV solution. See step 10 above if it is not.

20. If the medication is compatible, attach the secondary set to the secondary port on the primary line and secure it with adhesive tape.

21. Open the clamp on the secondary line and regulate it in accordance with the recommended rate for that medication.

    a. For continuous infusion set the secondary solution to the appropriate drip rate for the medication and then adjust the primary solution to achieve the desired total infusion flow.

    b. For intermittent infusion adjust the primary drip rate after the secondary solution is completed.

22. Record the IV infusion and medication.

23. Carefully monitor the IV infusion to maintain delivery of the medication and the IV fluid at the specified rate.

24. Assess the client's response to the medication in terms of the intended action of the medication, adverse reactions to it, discomfort, etc.

25. When the medication has infused, readjust the flow of the primary line at the correct rate.

PROCEDURE 44-12 **Administering Medication by IV Push**

An IV push (bolus) is the intravenous administration of a medication that cannot be diluted or that is needed in an emergency. Also, some drugs are administered this way to achieve maximum effect. It is important to remember that the medication is administered rapidly with an IV push, and this could be dangerous for the client. Some agencies allow only physicians or specially prepared nurses to administer IV push medications. Check agency policy.

An IV push can be administered directly into a vein through venipuncture, into an existing intravenous apparatus through an injection port (see Figure 44-6), or through an intermittent infusion set (*heparin lock*) when the client does not have an IV running but does have a heparin lock in place. The heparin lock, also referred to as a male adapter plug (MAP), is primarily used for clients who require regular intermittent IV medications but not the fluid volume of an intravenous infusion. The set usually consists of an indwelling needle or catheter attached to a plastic tube with a sealed injection tip. See Figure 44-7. It is called a heparin lock because small amounts of heparin are injected into it to maintain its patency. The infusion set is generally inserted into a client's arm or hand.

EQUIPMENT

- The physician's order or the medication card.
- The correct sterile medication.
- A sterile syringe of the appropriate size for the volume of medication and a sterile 2.5-cm (1-in.) #25 gauge needle to prevent large puncture holes in the injection port.
- Alcohol swabs.

In addition, for a heparin lock:

- A sterile syringe and needle with a heparin flush solution. Check agency practice. Many hospitals advocate the use of 100 units/mL of solution, and 0.5 mL is generally used. Prepackaged heparin syringes and needles are available.
- A sterile syringe and needle with 4 mL (or amount prescribed by the agency) of normal saline.

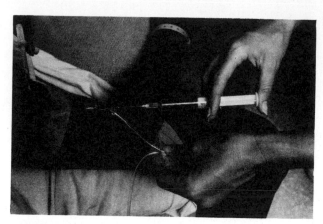

Figure 44-6
Administering medication through an injection port of an existing IV apparatus.

INTERVENTION

1. Check the physician's order carefully for the medication, dosage, route, and rate of administration.

   Rationale A medication that is injected too rapidly can create toxic concentrations in the blood plasma.

2. Prepare the medication according to Procedure 44-2 in *Introduction to Nursing*. Label the syringe with the name of the medication and the dosage.

3. In a separate syringe, prepare the heparin solution according to agency practice, if needed. Label this syringe. A prepackaged heparin syringe may be used.

4. In another syringe, prepare the saline solution. Label this syringe.

IV Push into an Existing IV

5. Inspect the injection site for any signs of infiltration, then identify an injection port nearest the client. Some ports have a circle indicating the site for the needle insertion.

   Rationale An injection port must be used because it is self-sealing. Any puncture to the plastic tubing will leak.

6. Clean the port with an antiseptic swab.

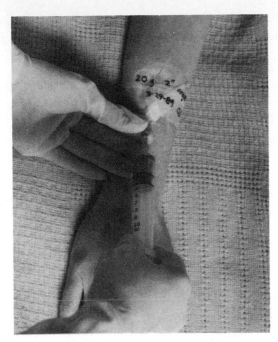

Figure 44–7
Administering medication through an intermittent
infusion set (heparin lock).

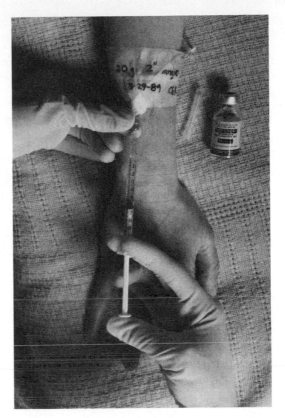

Figure 44–8

7. Stop the IV flow by closing the clamp or pinching
   the tubing above the injection port (see Figure
   44–6).

8. While holding the port steady, insert the needle
   into the port.

9. Draw back on the plunger to withdraw some blood
   into the IV tubing (not into the syringe).

   Rationale   This shows that the needle or catheter is in the vein.

10. Inject the medication at the ordered rate, with-
    draw the needle, reopen the clamp, and reestab-
    lish the intravenous infusion at the correct rate.
    If the medication is particularly irritating to the
    veins, run the IV rapidly for about a minute to
    dilute the medication, and then adjust the rate.

IV Push into an Intermittent Infusion Set (Heparin Lock)

11. Swab the injection port with an antiseptic swab.

12. Insert the needle with the normal saline into the
    port and aspirate for blood return. See Figure
    44–7.

    Rationale   This ensures that the heparin lock
    catheter is in the vein. In some situations blood
    will not return even though the heparin lock is
    patent.

13. Inject 2 mL of the normal saline solution. This
    step is optional. Check agency practice.

    Rationale   This is done to flush the heparin from
    the catheter and to verify patency of the vein. If
    the client experiences burning or stinging sen-
    sations, this may be normal or it may be that the
    needle or catheter is not in the vein and the fluid
    is infiltrating the tissue. In this case withhold the
    medication until the heparin lock is replaced.

14. Remove the saline-filled syringe, and cap the
    needle to maintain its sterility using the CDC
    approved method.

    Rationale   This syringe is used again, so it must
    be kept sterile.

15. Insert the needle attached to the medication
    syringe.

16. Inject the medication slowly at the recom-
    mended rate of infusion. Observe the client closely
    for adverse reactions. Remove the needle and
    syringe when all medication is administered.

17. Reattach the saline syringe, and inject the rec-
    ommended amount of saline.

    Rationale   The saline injection flushes the med-
    ication through the catheter and prepares the lock

for the heparin. Heparin is incompatible with many medications.

18. Insert the heparin syringe, and inject the heparin slowly into the set. See Figure 44–8.

19. Check the patency of the heparin lock at least every 8 hours or according to agency practice.

    a. Aspirate for return blood flow.

    b. Flush the catheter with 2–3 mL of normal saline.

    c. Refill the heparin lock with new heparin solution.

20. Check agency practice about recommended times for changing the heparin lock. Some agencies advocate a change every 48–72 hours.

IV Push Directly in Vein

21. Perform a venipuncture.

22. Slowly inject the medication into the vein. The rate of the injection will vary according to the medication, the physician's order, and/or the manufacturer's directions. Many medications are injected slowly over a period of several minutes. Often medications are diluted in the syringe to decrease the concentration in the client. Agency policies vary. Check drug reference information.

23. Withdraw the needle, and apply pressure to the site to prevent bleeding.

For All Types of Intravenous Medications

24. Document the medication given, dosage, time, route, all assessments, and your signature.

25. Carefully assess the client's response to the medication in terms of the intended action of the medication, adverse reactions to it, discomfort, etc.

PROCEDURE 44–13 **Administering Medications by Metered Dose Nebulizer**

A nebulizer is used to deliver a fine spray of medication into the nose or mouth. Nebulization is the production of a fog or mist. When the medication is intended for the nasal mucosa, it is inhaled through the nose; when it is intended for the trachea, bronchi, and/or lungs, it is inhaled through the mouth.

The metered dose nebulizer (see Figure 44–9), also called the hand nebulizer, is a container of medication that can be compressed by hand to release the medication through a nosepiece or mouthpiece. The force with which the air moves through the nebulizer causes the large particles of medicated solution to break up into finer particles, forming a mist or fine spray.

Many of the medications used to treat chronic obstructive pulmonary disease (COPD) or other respiratory problems are delivered through nebulization therapy. Common medications used are bronchodilators, mucolytic agents, antibiotics, and steroids.

EQUIPMENT

• Metered dose inhaler with medication cannister. This inhaler delivers a measured dose of drug with each push of the medication cannister, which fits into the top of the inhaler (see Figure 44–9).

INTERVENTION

1. When using oral metered dose nebulizers, clients need to be instructed to
   a. Place the mouthpiece of the inhaler into the mouth with its opening toward the throat or, with some models, to hold the mouthpiece 1–2 inches from the open mouth.
   b. Exhale through the nose as deeply as possible and then inhale slowly and deeply through the

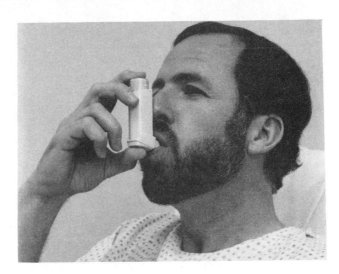

Figure 44–9
A metered dose, or hand, nebulizer.

mouth while releasing the dose. The dose is released by pressing down on the medication cannister.
   c. Hold the breath for several seconds to allow the aerosol to reach deeper branches of airways.
   d. Exhale slowly through pursed lips, which keeps the small airways open during exhalation.

2. When using inhalers, the client should be told to
   a. Breathe with normal force and depth.
   b. Release the medication while inhaling.

3. Caution all clients about overuse of the nebulizer since tolerance to the medication may occur and serious side effects result (eg, bronchospasm or adverse cardiac effects).

CHAPTER 45

WOUND CARE

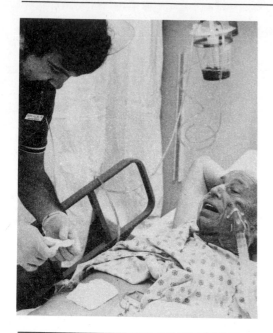

☐ The following procedures appear in *Introduction to Nursing:*

■ New procedures:

One of the functions of nurses is to promote wound healing, which may involve changing dressings, cleaning and shortening drains, and irrigating wound sites. Surgical aseptic technique is followed for most of these measures, to prevent the introduction of microorganisms into wounds.

PROCEDURE 45–8   **Applying a Stump Bandage**

When a limb is amputated, the distal portion of the limb that remains is called the stump. A stump bandage is usually applied to retain a dressing after a dressing change. It is also applied to apply pressure, support venous return flow, prevent swelling, and to help shape the stump. In some agencies, elasticized stump shrinkers are available to shape the stump in preparation for a prosthesis. See Figure 45–1.

If a stump shrinker is not available, determine the surgeon's preference regarding the type of material and the kind of bandage to apply. Some surgeons may request that the stump be wrapped with a figure-eight bandage; others prefer a recurrent or a spiral bandage. Commonly, the figure-eight or modified figure-eight bandages are used.

EQUIPMENT

- A clean bandage. The type of material will depend on the purpose of the bandage and the physician's order. An elastic bandage is often used to apply pressure. An 8-cm or 10-cm (3-in. or 4-in.) bandage is recommended for an adult's stump.

- Tape, safety pins, or metal clips to secure the bandage.

INTERVENTION

The following interventions describe bandaging a leg amputation; the bandaging of arm amputations is similar.

1. Obtain baseline assessment data.

2. Assist the client to a semi-Fowler's position in bed or to a sitting position on the edge of the bed.

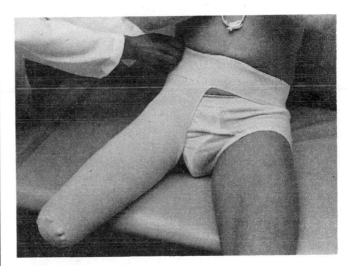

Figure 45–1
A stump shrinker.

3. For a figure-eight bandage:
   a. Anchor the bandage with two circular turns around the hips.
   b. Bring the bandage down over the stump and then back up and around the hips. See Figure 45–2.
   c. Bring the bandage down again, overlapping the previous turn, and make a figure eight around the stump and back up around the hips.
   d. Repeat, working the bandage up the stump. See Figure 45–3.
   e. Anchor the bandage around the hips with two circular turns.

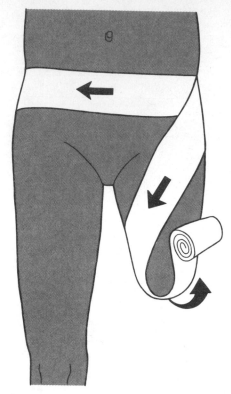

Figure 45–2

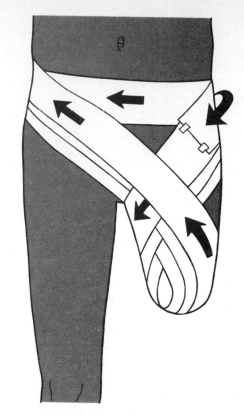

Figure 45–3

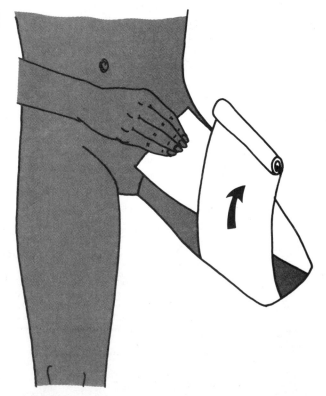

Figure 45–4

f. Secure the bandage with adhesive tape, safety pins, or clips.
or

g. Place the end of the elastic bandage at the top of the anterior surface of the leg and have the client hold it in place. Bring the bandage diagonally down toward the end of the stump.

h. Then, applying even pressure, bring the bandage diagonally upward toward the groin area. See Figure 45–4.

i. Make a figure-eight turn behind the top of the leg, downward again over and under the stump, and back up to the groin area. (See Figure 45–5.)

j. Repeat these figure-eight turns at least twice.

k. Anchor the bandage around the hips with two circular turns.

l. Secure the bandage with tape, safety pins, or clips.

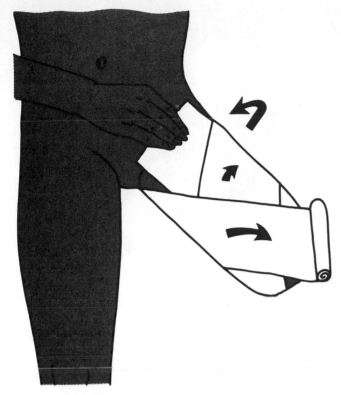

Figure 45–5

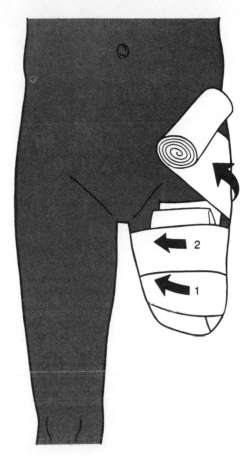

Figure 45–7

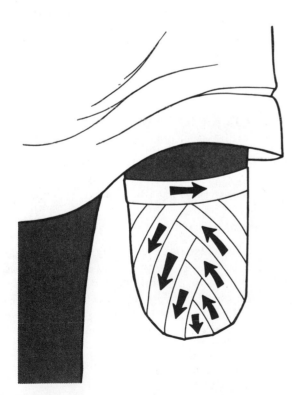

Figure 45–6

4. Recurrent bandage:
   a. Anchor the bandage with two circular turns around the stump.
   b. Cover the stump with recurrent turns.
   c. Anchor the recurrent bandage with two circular turns. See Figure 45–6.
   d. Secure the bandage with tape, safety pins, or clips.

5. Spiral bandage:
   a. Make recurrent turns to cover the end of the stump.
   b. Apply spiral turns from the distal aspect of the stump toward the body. See Figure 45–7.
   c. Anchor the bandage with two circular turns around the hips.
   d. Secure the bandage with tape, safety pins, or clips.

PROCEDURE 45-9 **Applying a Hot Water Bottle, Electric Heating Pad, or Aquathermia Pad**

A hot water bottle or bag is a common source of dry heat for local effect. It is convenient and relatively inexpensive. However, because there is a danger of burning from improper use, agencies may require the client to sign a release that absolves the agency and its employees from any responsibility for injury incurred with the use of hot water bottles.

Electric pads have become less popular in recent years. The pad provides a constant, even heat, is lightweight, and can be molded to a body part. Electric pads, however, can burn if the setting is too high. In some agencies the controls on the pads are set to a specific temperature to prevent burning.

The aquathermia, or aquamatic (water-flow), pad is becoming increasingly popular. Warm water circulates inside the pad, providing a controlled temperature.

Applications of heat are usually applied to

- Decrease muscle spasm and cramping
- Increase blood flow and enhance healing
- Reduce joint stiffness and increase joint range of motion
- Relieve pain
- Promote a feeling of comfort and relaxation

EQUIPMENT

Hot water bottle (bag):

- A hot water bottle with a stopper. Hot water bottles are usually made of plastic or rubber.
- A cover for the bottle. Some agencies have special covers; others use a soft towel.
- Hot water and a thermometer to measure the temperature of the water.

Electric heating pad:

- The electric pad and the control. Note whether the control is set at a specific temperature. Inspect the pad to make sure it is functioning correctly. A plastic key may be needed to set the temperature.
- A cover. Some electric pads have waterproof covers, which should be used if there will be moisture under the pad when it is applied.

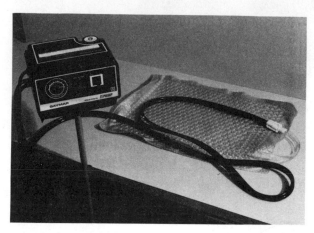

Figure 45-8
An aquathermia heating unit.

Aquathermia pad:

- The pad. Inside the pad are tubes containing distilled water.
- The control unit, which is operated by electricity. This unit has an opening, into which the water is poured, and a temperature gauge. The control unit is connected to the pad by tubing. See Figure 45-8.
- Distilled water for the unit.
- A cover for the pad. Some aquathermia pads have an absorbent surface through which moist heat can be applied. The other surface of the pad is waterproof. These pads are disposable.

Commercial hot packs:

- Dry heat can also be supplied by commercial packs. See Figure 45-9. They deliver a specific amount of heat for a specific time period. To start the heat, the pack is struck sharply or kneaded, which initiates a chemical reaction. Read the manufacturer's instructions before using the pack.

INTERVENTION

1. Obtain baseline assessment data.
2. Fold down the bedclothes to expose the area to which the heat will be applied.

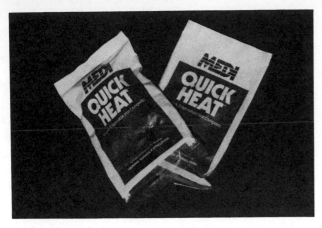

Figure 45–9
Commercially prepared disposable hot packs.

Hot Water Bottle

3. Fill the hot water bottle about two-thirds full.

4. Measure the temperature of the water if this was not done before the bag was filled. Follow agency practice for the appropriate temperature. Temperatures commonly used are

    a. 52 C (125 F) for a normal adult.

    b. 40.5–46 C (105–115 F) for a debilitated or unconscious adult.

    c. 40.5–46 C (105–115 F) for a child under 2 years of age.

5. Expel the air from the bottle.

    Rationale   Air remaining in the bottle prevents it from molding to the body part being treated.

6. Secure the stopper tightly.

7. Hold the bottle upside down and check for leaks.

8. Dry the bottle.

9. Wrap the bottle in a towel or hot water bottle cover.

10. Apply the bottle to the client. Support it against the body part with pillows as necessary.

11. Every 5–10 minutes, assess the client for any complaints of discomfort, eg, pain, burning, and skin reaction. Frequency of assessment depends on such factors as the client's previous responses to applications and ability to report problems. At the first sign of pain, swelling, or excessive redness, remove the heat and report any sign to the nurse in charge.

12. When the heat is applied, record the application, its purpose, the time, the method used, the site, and any nursing assessments.

13. Remove the heat before the rebound phenomenon begins, ie, 20–30 minutes. A hot water bottle will usually stay hot for the duration of the treatment. It needs to be replaced for the next application. If a disposable hot pack is used, the manufacturer's instructions state the length of time that heat is produced.

14. After removal, record the time and all nursing assessments.

Electric Heating Pad

15. Ensure that the body area is dry.

    Rationale   Electricity in the presence of moisture can conduct a shock.

16. Caution the client against inserting any sharp, pointed object, eg, a pin, into the pad.

    Rationale   A pin might strike a wire, damaging the pad and giving an electric shock to the client.

17. Place the cover on the pad. Some models have waterproof covers to be used when the pad is placed over a moist dressing.

    Rationale   Moisture could cause the pad to short circuit and burn or shock the client.

18. Plug the pad into the electric socket.

19. Set the control dial for the correct temperature. After the pad has heated, apply it to the body area. Follow steps 11–14.

Aquathermia Pad

20. Fill the unit with distilled water until it is two-thirds full. The unit will warm the water, which circulates through the pad.

21. Remove air bubbles and secure the top.

22. Regulate the temperature with the key if it has not been preset. Check the manufacturer's instructions.

23. Put the cover over the pad.

24. Plug in the unit.

25. Apply the pad to the body part. Follow steps 11–14.

| PROCEDURE 45–10 | **Applying a Heat Lamp or Heat Cradle** |

A heat lamp is often a gooseneck lamp with a special bulb or a 60-watt bulb in it. Also used is the infrared lamp, which has an infrared element rather than a bulb. Both lamps provide dry heat to a localized area.

A heat cradle is a metal frame that is placed on the bed over the client. It has a row of 25-watt light bulbs and provides less localized dry heat than a heat lamp.

Heat lamps and cradles are an effective means of applying heat to the skin without direct contact. This is important for clients who have painful wounds or sensitive skin conditions. Heat lamps or cradles are used to promote drying of draining wounds and to increase circulation to injured tissues.

EQUIPMENT

- A heat lamp or infrared lamp
or
- A heat cradle and bath blanket or sheet to cover the cradle

INTERVENTION

1. Obtain baseline assessment data.

Heat Lamp

2. Expose the area to be treated, and drape the client so that the body is exposed minimally.

3. Warn the client not to touch the bulb or element of the heat lamp.

4. Dry the area with a towel to remove all moisture.
   Rationale The skin is more likely to burn if moist.

5. Plug in the lamp, and place it the correct distance from the area to receive the heat. Direct the lamp carefully. A 60-watt bulb is usually placed 45–60 cm (18–24 in.) from the area being treated. Infrared lamps come in two sizes. Place a small lamp closer to the client, ie, 45–60 cm (18–24 in.) away. Place a large lamp 60–75 cm (24–30 in.) from the client. Do not cover the lamp.
   Rationale A cover on the lamp may catch fire.

6. Note and record the time that the treatment started.

7. Return every 5–10 minutes to assess the client.

8. Assess the client's discomfort and the appearance of the skin, eg, excessive redness. If unexpected reactions occur, turn off the heat and report the signs to the nurse in charge.

9. Remove the lamp at the designated time. Most treatments are ordered for 15–20 minutes. Dress any open area as required.

10. Document the treatment, the time, the length of the treatment, and nursing assessments.

Heat Cradle

11. Fold the top bedclothes to the bottom of the bed to make room for the cradle.

12. Warn the client not to touch the bulbs of the heat cradle.

13. Place the cradle carefully over the area to be heated.

14. Plug in the cradle, and check that the bulbs are on.

15. Cover the cradle with a bath blanket or sheet.
    Rationale The cover holds in the heat and prevents cooling by the circulating air.

16. Follow steps 6–10.

PROCEDURE 45–11 **Administering Hot Soaks and Sitz Baths**

A soak refers either to immersing a body part, eg, an arm, in a solution or to wrapping a part in gauze dressings and then saturating the dressing with a solution. Soaks may employ clean technique or sterile technique. Sterile technique is generally indicated for any open wounds, eg, a burn or an area that has had surgery. Dry dressings are usually applied between the soaks.

A sitz bath, or hip bath, is used to soak the client's pelvic area. The person sits in a special tub or chair, usually immersed from the midthighs to the iliac crests or umbilicus. Special tubs or chairs are preferred to the regular bathtub, which immerses the legs and results in less effective blood circulation to the perineum or pelvic area. See Figure 45–10. Disposable sitz baths are also available; they are commonly used in homes but may also be used in hospitals.

The order usually specifies the soak, its site, the type of solution, the temperature of the solution, the length of time for the soak, the frequency, and the purpose. Whether sterile technique is used is usually a nursing judgment; if there is a break in the skin, sterile technique is indicated. The duration of soaks is generally 15–20 minutes.

Soaks and sitz baths are generally administered

- To hasten suppuration, soften exudates, and enhance healing

- To apply medications to a designated area

- To clean a wound in which there is sloughing tissue or an exudate

- To promote circulation and enhance healing

EQUIPMENT

- A container such as a small basin to soak a finger or hand, a special arm or foot bath, or a sitz tub or chair.

- The specified solution at the correct temperature. If a temperature is not ordered, check agency policy; 40–43 C (105–110 F) is usually indicated, as tolerated by the client. Fill the container at least one-half full.

- A thermometer to test the temperature of the solution. Some sitz tubs have temperature indicators attached to the water taps.

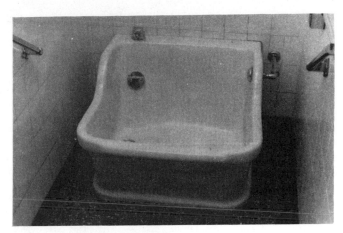

Figure 45–10
A sitz bath used in hospitals.

- Towels to support the limb against the sharp edge of a basin and to dry the body part following the soak.

- The required dressing materials. Gauze squares and roller gauze may be necessary following an extremity soak; perineal pads and a T-binder may be needed following a perineal soak.

- A bath blanket to wrap around the shoulders of a client during a sitz bath.

- A moisture-resistant bag for discarded dressings.

- Disposable gloves for the nurse if the client has any open areas on the skin.

INTERVENTION

1. Obtain baseline assessment data.

Hand or Foot Soak

2. Assist the client to a well-aligned, comfortable position to prevent muscle strain; the position adopted will be maintained for 15–20 minutes.

3. Don gloves as required, and remove the dressings, if any, and discard in the bag. Assess the amount, color, odor, and consistency of the drainage on removed dressings.

4. Pad the edge of the container with a towel, and immerse the body part in the container.

Rationale Padding is necessary to prevent pressure on the body part that rests on the edge of the container.

5. If the soak is sterile, cover the open container with a sterile drape or the container wrapper.

   Rationale Covering the open container helps prevent accidental contamination.

6. Maintain the temperature of the soak by placing a large sheet or blanket over the soak.

7. Assess the client and test the temperature of the solution at least once during the soak. Assess for discomfort, need for additional support, and any reactions to the soak. Report any unexpected responses to the nurse in charge immediately and terminate the soak. If the solution has cooled, remove the body part, empty the solution, add newly heated solution, and reimmerse the body part.

8. Remove the body part from the basin at completion of the soak, and dry it thoroughly. If the soak was sterile, use a sterile towel for drying.

9. Assess the appearance of the body part carefully, and reapply a dressing if required.

10. Document the soak, including duration, temperature, and type of solution. Note nursing assessments, including the appearance of the wound.

Sitz Bath

11. Fill the sitz bath with water at about 40 C (105 F). The water level in a tub should be at the umbilicus.

12. Pad the tub or chair with towels as required.

    Rationale Padding prevents pressure on the sacrum or posterior aspects of the thighs. When a disposable sitz bath on the toilet is used, a footstool can prevent pressure on the back of the thighs.

13. Remove the gown, or fasten it above the waist.

14. Don gloves if an open area or drainage is present.

15. Remove the T-binder and perineal dressings, if present, and note the amount, color, odor, and consistency of any drainage.

16. Assess the appearance of the area to be soaked for redness, swelling, odor, breaks in the skin, and drainage.

17. Wrap the bath blanket around the client's shoulders.

    Rationale The bath blanket will provide warmth.

18. Assist the client into the bath, and provide support for the client as needed. Leave a signal light within reach. Stay with the client if warranted, and terminate the bath as necessary.

    Rationale Some clients who have just had surgery or are weak may become faint or dizzy and need to be able to call a nurse or have the nurse remain with them.

19. Assess the client during the bath in terms of discomfort, color, and pulse rate. An accelerated pulse or extreme pallor may precede fainting. Immediately report any unexpected or adverse responses to the nurse in charge.

20. Test the temperature of the solution at least once during the bath. Adjust the temperature as needed.

21. Assist the client out of the sitz bath, and dry the area with a towel.

22. Assess the perineal area, and reapply dressings and garments as required.

23. Document the soak, including the duration, temperature, and type of solution. Note nursing assessments, including appearance of the wound.

Sample Recording

Date	Time	Notes
12/5/89	0900	43 C saline soak to (L) index finger × 20 min. 2 × 2 gauze saturated with purulent exudate. Finger measures 7 cm (down 1 cm from previous measurement) but continues to be red in color. ————————Toby N. Zacharias, NS

PROCEDURE 45-12   **Applying an Ice Bag, Ice Collar, Ice Glove, or Disposable Cold Pack**

The ice bag, a common device used in many homes and hospitals, is a moderate-sized rubber or plastic bag, into which pieces of ice can be inserted. The bag has a removable cap. Commercially prepared ice bags are available in some agencies. These bags are filled with an alcohol-based solution and sealed; they are kept in freezing units in a central supply area.

An ice collar is similar to an ice bag but is long and narrow. It is designed for use around the neck, though it can be used for other areas of the body. Commonly, it is used to control bleeding after a tonsillectomy.

The ice glove is simply a rubber or plastic glove that is filled with ice chips and tied at the open end. Gloves are generally used for small body parts, eg, an eye.

Disposable cold packs are similar to disposable hot packs. They come in a variety of sizes and shapes and provide a specific degree of coldness for a specified period of time, as indicated on the package. By striking, squeezing, or kneading the package, chemical reactions are activated that release the cold. The manufacturer's instructions must be followed. Most commercially prepared cold packs have soft outer coverings so they can be applied directly to the body part. See Figure 45-11.

Cold applications are generally applied

- To relieve headaches caused by vasodilation

- To prevent swelling of tissues and pain immediately following an injury or surgery

- To prevent, decrease, or terminate bleeding following an injury or surgery

EQUIPMENT

- An ice bag, collar, glove, or cold pack

- Ice chips

- A protective covering

- Roller gauze, a binder or a towel, and tape or safety pins to attach the device and keep it in place

- Disposable cold pack as required

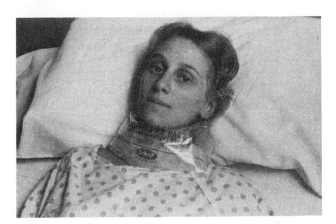

Figure 45-11
A disposable ice collar.

INTERVENTION

1. Assist the client to a comfortable position, and support the body part requiring the application.

2. Expose only the area to be treated, and provide warmth to avoid chilling. Privacy may or may not be necessary, depending on the location of the application and the client's wishes.

3. Obtain baseline assessment data.

Ice Bag, Collar, or Glove

4. Fill the device one-half to two-thirds full of crushed ice.
   Rationale   Partial filling makes the device more pliable so that it can be molded to a body part.

5. Remove excess air by bending or twisting the device.
   Rationale   Air inflates the device so that it cannot be molded to the body part.

6. Insert the stopper securely into an ice bag or collar, or tie a knot at the open end of a glove.
   Rationale   This prevents leakage of fluid when the ice melts.

7. Hold the device upside down and check it for leaks.

8. Cover the device with a soft cloth cover, if it is not already equipped with one.

   Rationale   The cover absorbs moisture that condenses on the outside of the device. It is also more comfortable for the client.

9. Apply the device for the time specified. The device is usually applied for no longer than 30 minutes because of the rebound phenomenon.

10. Hold it in place with roller gauze, a binder, or a towel. Secure with tape or safety pins as necessary.

11. Assess the client in terms of comfort and skin reaction (eg, pallor, mottled appearance, etc) as frequently as necessary for the client's safety, eg, every 5–10 minutes. Factors such as previous responses to applications and the client's ability to report any problems need to be considered.

12. At the time of application, document the cold application, its purpose, the method used, the site, and nursing assessments.

13. Remove the cold application at the designated time.

    Rationale   This avoids the harmful effects of prolonged cold.

14. After removal, record the time and assessments.

Disposable Cold Pack

15. Strike, squeeze, or knead the cold pack according to the manufacturer's instructions.

    Rationale   The action activates the chemical reaction that produces the cold.

16. Cover with a soft cloth cover if the pack does not have a cover. Most commercially prepared cold packs have soft outer coverings to permit application directly to the body part.

17. Follow steps 9–14.

PROCEDURE 45–13 **Administering a Cooling Sponge Bath**

The cooling sponge bath uses water or a combination of alcohol and water that is below body temperature. Alcohol evaporates at a low temperature and therefore removes body heat rapidly. However, alcohol-and-water sponge baths are less frequently used than in the past because alcohol has a drying effect on the skin. The temperatures for cooling sponge baths range from 18–32 C (65–90 F). A tepid sponge bath generally refers to one in which the water temperature is 32 C (90 F) throughout the bath. For a cool sponge bath, the water temperature is 32 C (90 F) at the beginning of the bath and is gradually lowered to 18 C (65 F) by adding ice chips during the bath. Cool sponge baths are used with extreme caution because of potential deleterious effects such as shock.

The purpose of a cooling sponge bath is to reduce a client's fever by promoting heat loss through conduction and vaporization. The decision to give a tepid sponge bath is generally made only after a marked fever is noted or a temperature increase of 1–2 C or 2–3 F. In some agencies a physician's order is required; others permit a decision by the nurse in charge.

EQUIPMENT

- A basin for the solution.
- A bath thermometer to check the temperature of the solution.
- A solution at the correct temperature. Water or equal portions of 70% alcohol and water are used.
- Ice chips for a cool sponge bath.
- Several washcloths and bath towels. Fewer are needed if ice bags or cold packs are used.
- A bath blanket.
- A thermometer to measure the client's temperature.
- A fan is sometimes used to increase air movement around the client, which lowers the body temperature through convection. In this case, drafts are not usually eliminated during the sponge bath.

INTERVENTION

1. If not already recorded prior to the sponge bath, measure the client's body temperature, pulse, and respirations to provide comparative baseline data.

Assess the client for other signs of fever: skin warmth, flushing, complaints of heat or chilling, diaphoresis, irritability, restlessness, general malaise, or delirium.

2. Explain that the face, arms, legs, back, and buttocks will be sponged, but not the chest and abdomen. The procedure takes about 30 minutes.

3. Remove the gown and assist the client to a comfortable supine position. Place a bath blanket over the client.

4. First sponge the client's face with plain water only, and dry it. An ice bag or cold pack may be applied to the head for comfort.

5. If ice bags or cold packs are not used, place bath towels under each axilla and shoulder.

   Rationale Bath towels protect the lower bed sheet from getting wet.

6. Wet three washcloths, wring them out so that they are very damp but not dripping, and place them in the axillae and groins. Or place ice bags or cold packs in these areas.

   Rationale Washcloths need to be as moist as possible to be effective. The axillae and groins contain large superficial blood vessels, which aid the transfer of heat.

7. Leave the washcloths in place for about 5 minutes, or until they feel warm. Rewet and replace them as required during the bath.

   Rationale Washcloths warm up relatively quickly in such vascular areas.

8. Place a bath towel under one arm. Sponge the arm slowly and gently for about 5 minutes or as tolerated by the client. Or place a saturated towel over the extremity, and rewet it as necessary. Give the client enough time to adjust to the initial reaction of chilliness and for the body to cool.

   Rationale Slow, gentle motions are indicated because firm rubbing motions increase tissue metabolism and heat production. Cool sponges given rapidly or for a short period of time tend to increase the body's heat production mechanisms by causing shivering.

9. Dry the arm, using a patting motion rather than a rubbing motion.

10. Repeat steps 8 and 9 for the other arm and the legs.

11. When sponging the extremities, hold the washcloth briefly over the wrists and ankles.

    Rationale The blood circulation is close to the skin surface in the wrists and ankles.

12. After 15 minutes check the client's vital signs. Compare with data taken before the bath.

    Rationale The vital signs are checked to evaluate the effectiveness of the sponge bath.

13. Ask the person to turn on his or her side, and sponge the back and buttocks for 3–5 minutes. Pat these areas dry.

14. Remove the washcloths or cold packs from the axillae and groins, and dry these areas.

15. Recheck the vital signs.

16. Document assessments, including the vital signs, as well as type of sponge bath given.

Sample Recording

Date	Time	Notes
12/5/89	1600	C/o headache, appears restless, is flushed and diaphoretic. T 104, P 110, R 24. Tepid sponge given.————
	1615	T 102, P 105, R 22. Is less restless. Headache, flushing and diaphoresis continue.————
	1630	T 100, P 100, R 20. Sponge bath discontinued. States headache "almost gone." No flushing or diaphoresis.——————————————Marya A. Shapiro, NS

PROCEDURE 45–14   **Applying a Moist Transparent Wound Barrier**

Transparent wound barriers such as Op-Site, Tega-derm, and Bio-occlusive are often applied to ulcerated or burned skin areas. Advantages of these dressings include

- They are nonporous, self-adhesive dressings that do not require changing as other dressings do. They are often left in place until healing has occurred or as long as they remain intact.

- Because they are transparent, the wound can be assessed through them.

- Because they are occlusive, the wound remains moist and retains the serous exudate, which hastens healing and reduces the risk of infection.

- Because they are elastic, they can be placed over a joint without disrupting the client's mobility.

- They adhere only to the skin area around the wound and not to the wound itself, because the wound is kept moist.

- They allow the client to shower or bathe without removing the dressing.

EQUIPMENT

- Soap and water to clean the surrounding skin area.

- A razor (optional) to shave the surrounding area.

- Alcohol or acetone to defat the surrounding skin.

- The wound barrier.

- Sterile gauze and the wound-cleaning agents specified by the physician or agency, eg, sterile saline, hydrogen peroxide, or Betadine. Check agency practice.

- Sterile gloves to wear when cleaning the wound.

- Scissors.

- Paper tape.

- A sterile #26 gauge needle and syringe to aspirate excessive drainage, if necessary.

INTERVENTION

1. If the size of the wound necessitates it, acquire the assistance of a coworker to help apply the dressing.

2. Thoroughly clean the skin area around the wound with soap and water. Shave the hair about 5 cm (2 in.) around the wound area if indicated. Then rub the area with alcohol or acetone, and allow it to dry.
   Rationale   Alcohol or acetone defats the skin. Defatted and clean, dry skin ensures better adhesion of the dressing.

3. Don sterile gloves, and clean the wound with the prescribed solution if indicated.

4. Assess the wound.

5. Remove part of the paper backing on the dressing. If you have an assistant, remove all of the paper backing; the two of you should hold the colored tabs attached to the dressing.

6. Apply the dressing at one edge of the wound site, allowing at least 2.5 cm (1 in.) coverage of the skin surrounding the wound.

7. Gently lay or press the barrier over the wound. Keep it free of wrinkles but avoid stretching it too tightly.
   Rationale   A stretched dressing restricts mobility.

8. Cut off the colored tabs after the wound is completely covered.

9. Remove gloves and discard.

10. Reinforce the edges of the dressing with paper or other porous tape.

11. Assess the wound at least daily to determine the extent of serous fluid accumulation under the dressing, wound healing, and the need to repair the dressing. For assessment of wound healing, see Procedure 45–3, step 3, in *Introduction to Nursing*.

12. If excessive serum has accumulated, use a #26 gauge needle to aspirate the fluid. Then patch the needle hole.

13. If the dressing is leaking, remove it and apply another dressing.

PROCEDURE 45–15 **Cleaning a Drain Site and Shortening a Penrose Drain**

Frequently, flexible rubber drains called *Penrose drains* are inserted during abdominal surgery to provide drainage of excessive serosanguineous fluid and purulent material and promote healing of underlying tissues by obliterating dead space. These drains may be inserted and sutured through the incision line, but they are most commonly inserted through stab wounds a few centimeters away from the incision line, so that the incision is kept dry. Without a drain, some wounds would heal over on the surface and trap the discharge inside. Then the tissues under the skin could not heal because of the discharge, and an abscess might form.

Drains vary in length and width. The length inserted can be 25–33 cm (10–14 in.), and the width 2.5–4 cm (0.5–1.5 in.). To facilitate drainage and healing of tissues from the inside to the outside or from the bottom to the top, the physician commonly orders that the drain be pulled out or shortened 2–5 cm (1–2 in.) each day. When a drain is completely removed, the remaining stab wound usually heals within 1–2 days. In some agencies this shortening procedure is performed only by physicians; in others, it is ordered by the physician and performed by nurses. Shortening of a drain is done in conjunction with a dressing change.

EQUIPMENT

- A sterile dressing set, including:
  - Gauzes for cleaning the wound.
  - A container for the cleaning solution.
  - A towel or drape.
  - Surgipads and/or gauze dressings.
  - Antiseptic solution.
  - Two pairs of forceps, including at least one hemostat.
- Cotton-tipped applicators.
- Sterile dressing materials sufficient to cover the surgical incision and the drain site. At least two 4 × 4 gauzes are usually needed to dress the drain site; more are required if drainage is copious. A sterile precut gauze is needed to apply first around the drain site.
- Sterile suture scissors if the drain has *not* been shortened previously. Drains that have not been shortened previously are attached to the skin by a

suture. The suture must be removed before shortening the drain.
- Sterile scissors to cut the drain.
- A sterile safety pin. Add this to the sterile dressing set.
- Disposable gloves (optional) for removing a moist outer dressing. Sterile gloves for shortening the drain.
- A moistureproof bag to receive the old dressings.
- Tape, tie tapes, or other binding supplies.
- A mask for the nurse and one for the client, if necessary.

INTERVENTION

1. Confirm the physician's order that the drain is to be shortened by the nurse and the length it is to be shortened, eg, 2.5 cm (1 in.).

2. Inform the client that the drain is to be shortened and that this procedure should not be painful. Explain that there may be a pulling sensation for a few seconds when the drain is being drawn out before it is shortened.

3. Ask the client not to speak unnecessarily or touch the wound during the dressing change, so as not to contaminate the wound. If the client will likely want to talk, provide the person with a mask.

4. Follow Procedure 45–2, steps 1–18, in *Introduction to Nursing.*

   Rationale The incision is cleaned first, since it is considered cleaner than the drain site. Moist drainage facilitates the growth of resident skin bacteria around the drain.

Cleaning the Drain

5. Clean the skin around the drain site by swabbing in half or full circles from around the drain site outward, using separate swabs for each wipe. See Figure 45–12. Forceps may be used in the nondominant hand to hold the drain erect while cleaning around it. Clean as many times as necessary to remove the drainage.

6. Assess the amount and character of drainage, including odor, thickness, and color.

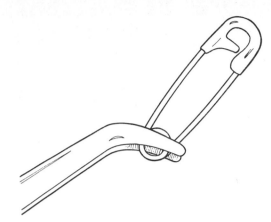

Figure 45-14

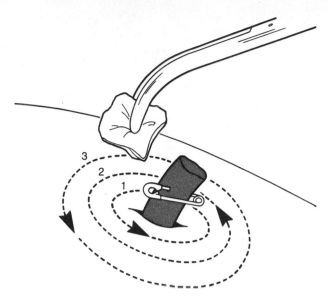

Figure 45-12

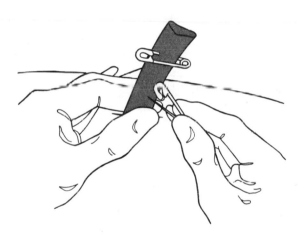

Figure 45-13

Shortening a Drain

7. If the drain has not been shortened before, cut and remove the suture. See Procedure 45-7 in *Introduction to Nursing*. The drain is sutured to the skin during surgery to keep it from slipping into the body cavity.

8. With a hemostat, firmly grasp the drain by its full width at the level of the skin, and pull the drain out the required length.

   Rationale   Grasping the full width of the drain ensures even traction.

9. Put on sterile gloves, and insert the sterile safety pin through the base of the drain as close to the skin as possible, holding the drain tightly against the skin edge and inserting the pin above your fingers. See Figure 45-13.

Rationale   The pin keeps the drain from falling back into the incision. Holding the drain securely in place at the skin level and inserting the pin above the fingers prevents the nurse from pulling the drain further out or pricking the client during this step.

or

Use two pairs of sterile forceps to shorten the drain. This procedure requires considerable manipulative skill.

a. After pulling the drain out, pick up the sterile safety pin at the clasp end by using one pair of forceps held in the nondominant hand.

b. Securely grasp the base of the pin with the hemostat held in the dominant hand. See Figure 45-14.

c. Holding the pin securely with the hemostat, open the pin by using the other forceps.

d. Use those forceps to hold the drain at the skin level while inserting the pin through the drain over the forceps.

e. Close the pin by using the forceps.

10. Cut off the excess drain so that about 2.5 cm (1 in.) remains above the skin. See Figure 45-15. Discard the excess in the waste bag.

11. Place a precut 4 × 4 gauze snugly around the drain (see Figure 45-16) or open a 4 × 4 gauze to 4 × 8, fold it lengthwise to 2 × 8, and place the 2 × 8 around the drain so that the ends overlap.

Rationale   This dressing absorbs the drainage and helps prevent it from excoriating the skin. Using precut gauze or folding it as described, instead of cutting the gauze, prevents any threads from coming loose and getting into the wound, where they could cause inflammation and provide a site for infection.

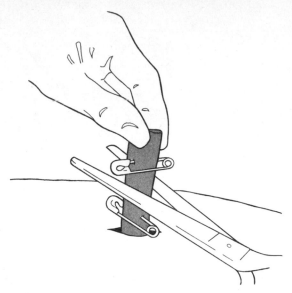

Figure 45–15

12. Apply the sterile dressings one at a time, using sterile gloved hands or sterile forceps. Take care that the dressings do not slide off and become contaminated. Place the bulk of the dressings over the drain area and below the drain, depending on the client's usual position.

    Rationale Layers of dressings are placed for best absorption of drainage, which flows by gravity.

13. Apply the final surgipad by hand, and secure the dressing with tape or ties.

14. Remove gloves and dispose of them.

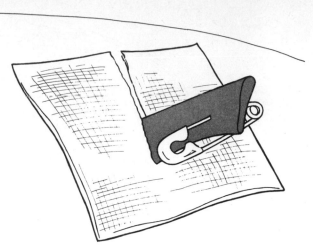

Figure 45–16

15. Document the procedure, including the amount the drain was shortened and the nursing assessments.

Sample Recording

Date	Time	Notes
12/5/89	1025	Penrose drain shortened 2.5 cm. Three 4 × 4 gauzes saturated with brownish yellow drainage. Dry dressings × 4 applied. Skin intact; no redness or irritation.———Maria L. Antonio, RN

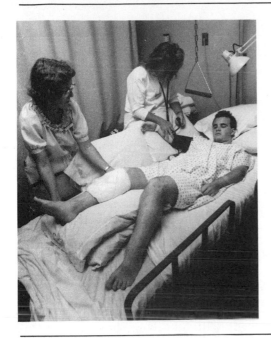

CHAPTER 46

PERIOPERATIVE CARE

☐ The following procedures appear in *Introduction to Nursing:*

Procedure 46–1
Teaching Moving, Leg Exercises, and Coughing and Deep-Breathing Exercises

Procedure 46–2
Inserting and Removing a Nasogastric Tube

Procedure 46–3
Making a Surgical Bed

Procedure 46–4
Measuring and Applying Antiemboli Stockings

Procedure 46–5
Managing Gastrointestinal Suction

■ New procedures:

Procedure 46–6
Performing a Surgical Hand Scrub

Procedure 46–7
Surgical Skin Preparation

Procedure 46–8
Initiating, Maintaining, and Terminating a Blood Transfusion

One aspect of preoperative care is preparing the skin prior to surgery. The Centers for Disease Control recommend that hair near the operative site not be removed unless absolutely necessary. If hair must be removed, clip it or use a depilatory rather than shaving it.

PROCEDURE 46–6 **Performing a Surgical Hand Scrub**

A surgical hand scrub is intended to render the skin of the hands as free of microorganisms as possible. It is performed by nurses employed in operating rooms, delivery rooms, burn units, and in special diagnostic areas. The scrub lasts 5–10 minutes, depending upon agency practice. Brushes or sponges and antimicrobial agents are employed to remove bacteria on the hands.

The exact technique for a surgical hand scrub varies among agencies. The practices that follow should be carried out before beginning the scrub.

1. Nails must be short, clean, and free of nail polish. Artificial nails should not be worn.

2. Hands and arms should be free of cuts, abrasions, and other problems.

3. The cap should be in place and completely cover all the hair.

4. The mask should be in place.

There are two types of surgical scrubs: the stroke-count scrub and the timed scrub. They both take about 5 minutes to complete. The stroke-count scrub involves a specific number of cleaning strokes for each aspect of the hands and arms. With the timed scrub each area is scrubbed for a specific length of time. The fingers and hands are scrubbed, then the arms to 5 cm (2 in.) above each elbow. Most agencies have specific recommended practices regarding the surgical hand scrub.

EQUIPMENT

- An antimicrobial solution. Most agencies supply a liquid antiseptic beside the sink. The container of antiseptic solution is often operated by a foot pedal. In some agencies, antimicrobial soap waters are available.

- A deep sink with foot, knee, or elbow controls for the water and a faucet high enough so that the hands and forearms can be positioned under it. See Figure 46–1.

- Towels for drying the hands. Many agencies supply sterile towels.

- A nail-cleaning tool, such as a file or orange stick.

- Two surgical scrub brushes. Some commercially prepared sponge brushes are impregnated with antimicrobial soap.

- Mask and cap.

INTERVENTION

1. Remove your wristwatch and rings. Ensure that your fingernails are trimmed.
   Rationale A wristwatch and rings can harbor microorganisms and be damaged by water.

2. Make sure that sleeves are above the elbows.
   Rationale The hands and lower arms are washed.

3. Ensure that your uniform is tucked in at the waist.
   Rationale A loose-fitting uniform can contaminate the hands if it touches them.

4. Apply cap and face mask.

5. Turn on the water and adjust the temperature to lukewarm.
   Rationale Warm water removes less protective oil from the skin than hot water. Soap irritates the skin more when hot water is used.

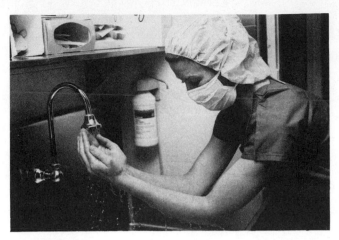

Figure 46–1

6. Wet the hands and forearms under running water, holding the hands above the level of the elbows so that the water runs from the fingertips to the elbows. See Figure 46–1.

   Rationale   The hands will become cleaner than the elbows. The water should run from the least contaminated to the most contaminated area.

7. Apply 2–4 mL (1 tsp) antiseptic solution to the hands.

8. Use firm, rubbing, circular movements to wash the palms and backs of the hands, the wrists, and the forearms. Interlace the fingers and thumbs, and move the hands back and forth. Continue washing for 20–25 seconds.

   Rationale   Circular strokes clean most effectively, and rubbing ensures a thorough mechanical cleaning action. (Other areas of the hands still need to be cleaned, however.)

9. Hold the hands and arms under the running water to rinse thoroughly, keeping the hands higher than the elbows.

   Rationale   Antiseptic remaining on the skin is irritating. The nurse rinses from the cleanest to the least clean area.

10. Check the nails, and clean them with a file or orange stick if necessary. Rinse the nail tool after each nail is cleaned.

Rationale   Sediment under the nails is removed more readily when the hands are moist. Rinsing the nail tool prevents the transmission of sediment from one nail to another.

11. Apply antiseptic solution and lather the hands again. Using a scrub brush, scrub each hand for 45 seconds. Scrub each side of all fingers including the skin between each finger and the thumb, and the back and the palm of the hand.

    Rationale   Scrubbing loosens bacteria, including those in the creases of the hands.

12. Using the scrub brush, scrub from the hands to 5 cm (2 in.) above each elbow. Scrub all sides of the arms for about 45 seconds while continuing to hold hands higher than the elbows.

    Rationale   Scrubbing is done from the cleanest area (hands) to the least clean area (upper arm).

13. Discard the brush.

14. Rinse hands and arms thoroughly so that the water flows from the hands to the elbows.

    Rationale   Rinsing removes resident and transient bacteria and sediment.

15. Turn off the water with the foot or knee pedal.

16. Use a sterile towel to dry one hand thoroughly, from the fingers to the elbow. Use a rotating motion. Use a second sterile towel to dry the second hand in the same manner. In some agencies towels are of a sufficient size that one half can be used to dry one hand and arm and the second half for the second hand and arm.

    Rationale   Moist skin readily becomes chapped and subject to open sores. Thorough drying also makes it easier to don sterile gloves. The nurse dries the hands from the cleanest to the least clean area.

17. Discard the towels.

18. Keep the hands in front of you and above your waist.

    Rationale   This position maintains the cleanliness of the hands and prevents accidental contamination.

PROCEDURE 46–7 **Surgical Skin Preparation**

The purpose of preparing the skin before surgery (preoperative skin preparation) is to destroy microorganisms and thus reduce the chance of infection.

It is recommended that the hair near the operative site not be removed unless absolutely necessary. In some agencies the client's skin is "prepped" in a special room just before surgery. If hair must be removed, the CDC recommend that it be removed with clippers or a depilatory and that the area be cleansed with antimicrobials just before surgery.

The area prepared is generally larger than the incision area. This practice minimizes the number of microorganisms in the areas adjacent to the incision. Hospital policy describes what area and how the skin is prepared before various operations.

The Association of Operating Room Nurses recommends that hair removal only be done as necessary. Studies have shown that the method of hair removal affects skin infection rates. One study showed an infection rate of 2.5% in clients shaved with an electric razor, whereas clients neither clipped nor shaved had an infection rate of 0.9%.

Prior to any skin preparation, it is important to carefully inspect the prospective surgical area for growths, moles, rashes, pustules, irritations, exudate, abrasions, bruises, or any broken or ischemic areas. These should be recorded and reported to the surgeon. In addition, the nurse must determine whether the client is allergic to any of the solutions used in the skin preparation, eg, iodine in the antiseptic.

EQUIPMENT

- Adequate lighting for clear visibility of the hair on the skin

- A bath blanket to drape the client

Clipping:

- Electric clippers with sharp heads and unbroken teeth

- Scissors for long hair, if needed

- Antimicrobial solution and applicators, if needed

Wet shave:

The CDC do not recommend wet shaving.

- Skin preparation set, which contains a disposable razor, compartmentalized basin for solutions, moistureproof drape to protect the bedding, soap solution, sponges for applying the soap solution, and cotton-tipped applicators for cleaning areas such as the umbilicus

- Warm water to make the soap solution

INTERVENTION

Before Clipping

1. Drape the client. Expose only the area to be clipped at one time. You will clip about 15 cm (6 in.) at a time.

Clipping

2. Make sure the area is dry.

3. Remove hair with clippers; do not apply pressure.
   Rationale Pressure can cause abrasions, particularly over bony prominences.

4. Move the drape, and repeat steps 2 and 3 until the entire area to be prepared is clipped. If applying antimicrobial solution, follow steps 10–11.

Wet Shaving

5. Place the moistureproof towel under the area to be prepared.

6. Lather the skin well with the soap solution.
   Rationale One research study showed that soaking the skin hair in lather for 4 minutes allows the keratin to absorb water and thereby makes the hair easier and softer to remove.

7. Stretch the skin taut and hold the razor at about a 45° angle to the skin. Shave in the direction in which the hair grows. Use short strokes and rinse the razor frequently.
   Rationale Rinsing removes hairs and lather that can obstruct the blade.

8. Wipe excess hair off the skin with the sponges.

9. Move the drape and repeat steps 6–8 until the entire area to be prepared is shaved.

Cleaning and Disinfecting

10. Clean any body crevices, such as the umbilicus, nails, and ear canals, with applicators and solutions. Dry with swabs.

11. If an antimicrobial solution is used, apply to the area immediately after it is clipped. Leave it for the designated time, then dry the area with clean swabs. Agency policy will guide you on whether to use an antimicrobial solution and, if so, which to use and how long to leave it on.

After Clipping

12. After clipping, the skin preparation may need to be checked by the nurse in charge. Report to the nurse in charge any abrasions, including those made by the clippers or razor.

13. Remove the waterproof towel and bath blanket carefully so as not to spill the clipped hairs onto the bed.

14. Document the skin preparation on the client's chart.

Sample Recording

Date	Time	Notes
12/5/89	0830	Hair clipped on left lower extremity. Skin intact. Appeared tense. Stated: "I hope the scar won't show much."————————————Eunice L. Lentz, NS

PROCEDURE 46–8 **Initiating, Maintaining, and Terminating a Blood Transfusion**

A *blood transfusion* is the introduction of whole blood or components of the blood—such as plasma, serum, erythrocytes, or platelets—into the venous circulation.

Transfusion reactions can be categorized as hemolytic, febrile, and allergic. The nurse must assess a client closely for reactions. Signs of an acute reaction include sudden chills or fever, low back pain, drop in blood pressure, nausea, flushing, agitation or respiratory disorders. Signs of less severe allergic reactions include hives and itching but no fever.

EQUIPMENT

- A unit of whole blood. Blood is usually provided in plastic bags by the blood bank. One unit of whole blood is 500 mL of blood in a container. No more than one blood component or unit is obtained for the client at a time.

- A blood administration set. There are two types: a straight line and a Y-set. The Y-set is preferred because the infusion can be maintained with saline if any adverse effects arise from the transfusion. In many instances, however, the tubing must also be changed. The infusion tubing has a filter inside the drip chamber. The tubing clamp should be just under the drip chamber. A Y-set can also be used when a saline solution is needed to run with the blood (eg, when giving packed cells) or to flush the line before the blood enters the tubing (eg, when running an IV infusion that is not saline).

- A venipuncture set containing a #18 needle or catheter, if one is not already in place, alcohol swabs, and tape. When blood is to be administered quickly, a #15 needle or a larger catheter, eg, #14, is often used. Large-gauge needles prevent damage to red blood cells (RBCs).

- A container of 250 mL of saline solution. Some agencies recommend that saline be run through the tubing before and after a blood transfusion.

- An IV pole.

- Gloves for the nurse.

INTERVENTION

1. Obtain the following assessment data:
   a. Baseline data about the client's blood pressure, pulse, temperature, and respirations, if data are not already available.
   b. Whether the client has known allergies or has had previous adverse reactions to blood.
   c. Specific signs related to the client's pathology and reason for needing the transfusion. For example, for an anemic client, note the hemoglobin level.

2. Determine that there is a signed consent form from the client, if required by the agency. If the client is a Jehovah's Witness, written permission is required.

3. If the client has an IV running, check whether the needle and solution are appropriate to administer blood. The needle should be #18 gauge or larger, and the solution must be saline. If the infusion is not compatible, remove it, and cap the bottle to maintain sterility. Dextrose, Ringer's solution, medications and other additives, and hyperalimentation solutions are incompatible.

4. When obtaining the blood, check the requisition form and the blood bag label with a laboratory technician or according to agency policy. Specifically check the client's name, identification number, blood type (A, B, AB, or O) and Rh group, the blood donor number, and the expiration date of the blood.

5. With another nurse (the agency may require an RN) compare the laboratory blood type record with
   a. The client's name and identification number. Ask the client to state his or her full name as a double check.
   b. The number on the blood bag label.
   c. The ABO group and Rh type on the blood bag label.

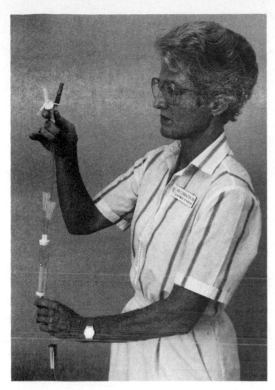

Figure 46–2

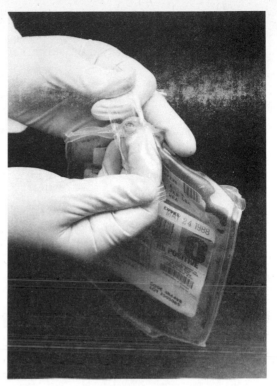

Figure 46–3

6. Sign the appropriate form with the other nurse according to agency policy.

7. Make sure that the blood is left at room temperature for no more than 30 minutes before starting the transfusion (RBCs deteriorate and lose their effectiveness after 2 hours at room temperature). Agencies may designate different times at which the blood must be returned to the blood bank if it has not been started. As blood components warm, the risk of bacterial growth also increases.

Initiating a Transfusion

If the client does not have an IV running, you need to perform a venipuncture on a suitable vein and start an IV infusion of normal saline. In some agencies an IV must be running before the blood is obtained from the blood bank.

8. Obtain a Y-set for blood administration. See Figure 46–2.

9. Ensure that the attached blood filter is suitable for whole blood or the blood components to be transfused. Blood filters have a surface area large enough to allow the blood components through easily but are designed also to trap clots.

10. Close all the clamps on the Y-set: the main flow rate clamp and both Y-line clamps.

11. Spike a container of 0.9% saline solution with the Y-set spike containing the vented tubing.

12. Invert the blood bag gently several times to mix the cells with the plasma.
    Rationale Rough handling can damage the cells.

13. Expose the port on the blood bag by pulling back the tabs. See Figure 46–3.

14. Insert the remaining Y-set spike into the blood bag.

15. Hang the saline solution and blood with the Y-set attached on an IV pole about 1 m (36 in.) above the planned venipuncture site.

16. Open the clamp on the normal saline tubing, and squeeze the drip chamber until it is ⅓ full.

17. Remove the IV tubing needle adaptor cover, open the main flow rate clamp, and prime the tubing.

Close both clamps and replace the needle adaptor cover.

18. Don gloves and perform a venipuncture if required.

19. Attach the primed infusion tubing to the IV needle and tape it securely.

20. Establish intravenous flow by opening the saline solution clamp and the main roller clamp.

21. Close the saline solution clamp and the main flow clamp and open the blood line clamp.

22. Squeeze the blood drip chamber until the filter is completely immersed in blood.

23. Open the main flow rate clamp and regulate the blood's flow rate.

24. Run the blood for the first 15 minutes at 20 drops per minute. Stay with and observe the client closely for the first 5–10 minutes. Note adverse reactions such as chilling, nausea, vomiting, skin rash, or tachycardia.

    Rationale The earlier a transfusion reaction occurs, the more severe it tends to be. Identifying such reactions promptly helps to minimize the consequences. Instruct the client to call you immediately if any unusual symptoms are felt during the transfusion.

25. If any of these reactions occur, close the clamp on the transfusion, open the clamp on the tubing with normal saline, and notify the nurse in charge or physician immediately. Follow agency procedure about obtaining urine specimens, etc.

26. Record starting the blood, including vital signs, type of blood, blood unit number, sequence number (eg, #1 of three ordered units), site of the venipuncture, size of the needle, and drip rate.

Maintaining a Transfusion

27. Fifteen minutes after initiating the transfusion, check the client's vital signs. If there are no signs of a reaction, establish the required flow rate. Most adults can tolerate receiving one unit of blood in 1½ to 2 hours.

28. Assess the client every 30 minutes, or more often, depending on the health status, including vital signs.

Terminating a Transfusion

29. Don gloves.

30. If no infusion is to follow, clamp the blood tubing and remove the needle.
    or
    If the primary IV is to be continued, flush the line with the saline solution, attach the primary IV container, and adjust the drip to the desired rate. Often a normal saline or other solution is kept running in case of a delayed reaction to the blood.

31. Discard the administration set according to agency practice. Needles should be placed in a labeled puncture-resistant container designated for such disposal. Blood bags and administration sets should be bagged and labeled before being sent for decontamination and processing. See agency policy.

32. Remove gloves.

33. Again monitor vital signs.

34. On the requisition attached to the blood unit, fill in the time the transfusion was completed and the amount transfused.

35. Attach one copy of the requisition to the client's record and another to the empty blood bag.

36. Return the blood bag and requisition to the blood bank.

37. Record completion of the transfusion, the amount of blood absorbed, the blood unit number, and the vital signs. If the primary IV infusion was continued, record connecting it.

Sample Recording

Date	Time	Notes
12/12/89	1100	1 unit whole blood administered. No adverse reactions. BP stable at 120/70, TPR 37, 88, 14. 500 mL saline started at 20 gtt/min. ——Selina L. Ward SN

BIBLIOGRAPHY

Acee S: Helping patients breathe more easily. *Geriatr Nurs* (July/August) 1984; 4:230−33.

Administering oxygen safely: When, why, how. *Nurs 80* (October) 1980; 10:54−56.

American Heart Association: *Recommendations for Human Blood Pressure Determination by Sphygmomanometers.* Pub No. 70-019-B, 80-100M, 9-81-100M. American Heart Association, 1980.

American Heart Association. Standards and guidelines for cardiopulmonary resuscitation (CPR) and emergency cardiac care (ECC). *JAMA* June 1986; 255:2905−84.

Anderson MA, Aker SN, Hickman RO: The double-lumen Hickman catheter. *Am J Nurs* (February) 1982; 82:272−73.

Axnick KJ, Yarbrough M (eds.): *Infection Control: An Integrated Approach.* Mosby, 1984.

Baker NC, Cerone SB, Gaze N, Knapp TR: The effect of type of thermometer and length of time inserted on oral temperature measurements of afebrile subjects. *Nurs Res* (March/April) 1984; 33:109−111.

Bates B: *A Guide to Physical Examination,* 4th ed. Lippincott, 1987.

Bayer LM, Scholl DE, Ford EG: Tube feeding at home. *Am J Nurs* (September) 1983; 83:1321−25.

Beck M: Patient education: Gastric tube feeding. *SGAJ* (Fall) 1985; 8:35−36.

Birdsall C, Ruggio J: Mouth-to-mouth resuscitation—Is there a safe, effective alternative? *Am J Nurs* (August) 1987; 87:1019.

Bowers AC, Thompson JM: *Clinical Manual of Health Assessment,* 3d ed. Mosby, 1988.

Bridge P, Carlson RA: Preadmission assessment of the elderly. *Canad Nurse* (December) 1983; 79:27−29.

Brogna L, Lakaszawski ML: The continent ostomy . . . the Kock pouch. *Am J Nurs* (February) 1986; 86:160−63.

Brozenec S: Caring for the postoperative patient with an abdominal drain. *Nurs 85* (April) 1984; 15:55−57.

Bruno P, Craven RF: Age challenges to wound healing. *J Gerontol Nurs* (December) 1982; 8(12):686−91.

Byrne CJ, Saxton DF, Pelikan PK, Nugent PM: *Laboratory Tests: Implications for Nursing Care,* 2d ed. Addison-Wesley, 1986.

Caring for a patient with a urinary diversion stoma. *Nurs 84* (July) 1984; 14:16−19.

Carroll M: Infection control in long-term care. *Geriatr Nurs* (March/April) 1984; 5:100−103.

Carroll PF: The ins and outs of chest drainage systems. *Nurs 86* (December) 16:26−34.

Centers for Disease Control: *Recommendations for prevention of HIV transmission in health care settings.* MMWR 1987 (suppl); 36:3s−18s.

Clayton M: The right way to prevent medication errors. *RN* (June) 1987; 50:30−1.

Cohen MR: Play it safe. Don't use these abbreviations. *Nursing* (July) 1987; 17:46−47.

Cohen MR: Use caution if you must administer medications obtained from a source other than the pharmacy. *Nursing* (January) 1984; 14:25. Canadian ed. 14:26.

The Committee on Transfusion Practices, American Association of Blood Banks: The latest protocols for blood transfusions. *Nurs 86* (October) 1986; 16:34−41.

D'Agostino JS: Set your mind at ease on oxygen toxicity. *Nurs 83* (July) 1983; 13:54−56.

Dalrymple D: Setting up for thoracic drainage. *Nurs 84* (June) 1984; 14:12−14.

Davis NM, Cohen MR: Learning from mistakes: medication errors to avoid. *Nursing* (May) 1987; 17:84, 87−88, 90.

DeYoung M: Planning for discharge. *Geriatr Nurs* (November/December) 1982; 3:396−99.

Drain CB: Managing postoperative pain . . . It's a matter of sighs. *Nurs 84* (August) 1984; 14:52−55.

Eliopoulos C, ed.: *Health Assessment of the Older Adult.* Addison-Wesley, 1984.

Erickson R: Tube talk. Principles of fluid flow in tubes. *Nurs 82* (July) 1982; 12:54–61.

Farrell J: *Illustrated Guide to Orthopedic Nursing*, 3d ed. Lippincott, 1986.

Flynn ME, Rovee DT: Wound healing mechanisms. *Am J Nurs* (October) 1982; 82:1544–50.

Fuchs PL: Getting the best out of oxygen delivery systems. *Nurs 80* (December) 1980; 10:34–43.

Fuchs PL: Streamlining your suctioning techniques, part 1: Nasotracheal suctioning. *Nurs 84* (May) 1984; 14:55–61.

Fuchs PL: Streamlining your suctioning techniques, part 3: Tracheostomy suctioning. *Nurs 84* (July) 1984; 14:39–43.

Garner JS, Favero MS: *Guidelines for handwashing and hospital environmental control.* U.S. Government Printing Office, 1985.

Garner JS, Simmons BP: CDC guidelines for isolation precautions in hospitals. *Infect Control* (July/August) 1983; 4:254–325.

Guyton AC: *Textbook of Medical Physiology*, 7th ed. Saunders, 1986.

Hahn AB, Barkin RL, and Oestreich SJK: *Pharmacology in Nursing*, 16th ed. Mosby, 1986.

Hudson B: Sharpen your vascular skills with the Doppler ultrasound stethoscope. *Nurs 83* (May) 1983; 13:55–57.

Huey FL: Setting up and troubleshooting. *Am J Nurs* (July) 1983; 83:1026–28.

Influencing repair and recovery. *Am J Nurs* (October) 1982; 82:1550–57.

Jackson J: "Don't shout, nurse!" . . . hearing problems in the elderly. *Geriatr Nurs* (May–June) 1986; 6:12–13.

Jackson MM: From ritual to reason—with a rational approach for the future: An epidemiologic perspective. Fifth Annual Carole DeMille Lecture. *Infect Control* (August) 1984; 12(4):213–220.

Jackson MM, Lynch P: Infection control: too much or too little?—Undiagnosed cases. *AJN* (February) 1984; 84:208–210.

Jackson MM, Lynch P: Isolation practices: a historical perspective. *Am J Infect Control* (February) 1985; 13:21–31.

Jackson MM, Lynch P, McPherson DC et al: Why not treat all body substances as infectious? *Am J Nurs* (September) 1987; 87:1137–39.

Jacobs L, Fontana R, Albert D: Is that geriatric patient really ready to go home? *RN* (November) 1985; 48:40–43.

Karrei I: Hickman catheters: Your guide to troublefree use. *Canad Nurse* (December) 1982; 78:25–27.

Keithley JK, Fraulini KE: What's behind that I.V. line? *Nurs 82* (March) 1982; 12:32–42.

Keithley JK, Tasic PW: A unified approach to assessment of the surgical patient. *Am J Nurs* (April) 1982; 82:612–14.

Killon A: Reducing the risk of infection from indwelling urethral catheters. *Nurs 82* (May) 1982; 12:84–88.

Kinney AB, Blount M, Dowell M: Urethral catheterization: Pros and cons of an invasive but sometimes essential procedure. *Geriatr Nurs* (November/December) 1980; 1:258–63.

Kneedler JA, Dodge GH: *Perioperative Patient Care: The Nursing Perspective*, Blackwell, 1983.

Kniep-Hardy MJ, Votava K, Stubbings MJ: Managing indwelling catheters in the home. *Geriatr Nurs* (October) 1985; 6:280–85.

Konstantinides NN, Shronts E: Tube feeding: Managing the basics. *Am J Nurs* (September) 1983; 83:1312–18.

Lane PL, Lee MM: New synthetic casts: What nurses need to know. *Orthop Nurs* (November/December) 1982; 1(6):13–20.

Lane PL, Lee MM: Special care for special casts. *Nurs 83* (July) 1983; 13(7):50–51.

Larson E: Bringing the new isolation guideline into focus. *Am J Infect Control* (December) 1984; 12(6):312–16.

Larson E: Current handwashing issues. *Infect Control* (January) 1984; 5(1):15–17.

Lehmann JF, DeLateur BJ: *Therapeutic Heat and Cold.* 3d ed. Williams and Wilkins, 1982.

Lewis CB: *Aging: The Health Care Challenge.* Davis, 1985.

Logio T: Suppository insertion—which end is first? *Nurs 85* (February) 1985; 15:10.

Luce JM, Tyler ML, and Pierson DJ: *Intensive Respiratory Care.* Saunders, 1984.

MacLean J, Shamian J, Butcher P: Restraining the elderly agitated patient. *Canad Nurs* (June) 1982; 68:44–46.

Magdziak BJ: There's just no excuse for IV complications. *RN* (February) 1988; 51:30–31.

Mager-O'Connor E: How to identify and remove fecal impactions. *Geriatr Nurs* (May/June) 1984; 5:158–61.

Malasanos L, Barkauskas V, Moss M, Stoltenberg-Allen K: *Health Assessment*, 3d ed. Mosby, 1986.

Metheny MM: 20 ways to prevent tube-feeding complications. *Nurs 85* (January) 1985; 15:47–50.

Miller J: Helping the aged manage bowel function. *J Gerontol Nurs* (February) 1985; 11:37–41.

Miller KS: Chest tubes: Indications, techniques, management and complications. *Chest* (February) 1987; 91:258–64.

Monahan FD: When swallowing pills is difficult. *Geriatr Nurs* (March/April) 1984: 5:88–89.

Moore MC: Do you still believe these myths about tube feeding? *RN* (May) 1987; 50:51–52, 54.

Mott SR, Fazekas NF, James SR: *Nursing Care of Children and Families: A Holistic Approach.* Addison-Wesley, 1985.

Munro-Black J: The ABC's of total parenteral nutrition. *Nurs 84* (February) 1984; 14:50–56.

National Heart, Lung, and Blood Institute: *The 1984 Report of the Joint National Committee on Detection, Evaluation, and Treatment of High Blood Pressure,* U.S. Department of Health and Human Services, Public Health Service, National Institutes of Health, 1984. Reprinted from *Arch Intern Med* (May) 1984; 144:1045–57.

The National Intravenous Therapy Association's intravenous nursing standards of practice: Home I.V. therapy. *J Natl IV Ther Assoc* (March/April) 1984; 7:93.

Neuberger GB: Wound care: What's clear what's not. *Nurs 87* (February) 1987; 17:34–37.

Northridge JAS: Helpful hints for assessing the ostomate. *Nurs 82* (April) 1982; 12:72–77 (Canadian ed. 12:8–13).

Nottebart HC: The CDC guidelines for prevention and control of nosocomial infections: View from the trenches. (Commentary.) *Am J Infect Control* (February) 1985; 13(1):40–44.

Osborne LJ, Digiacomo I: Traction: A review with nursing diagnoses and interventions. *Orthop Nurse* (July/August) 1987; 6:13–19.

Palau D, Jones S: Test your skill at trouble shooting chest tubes. *RN* (October) 1986; 49:43–45.

Palestis E: The admission ward concept. *Geriatr Nurs* (January/February) 1986; 7:40–41.

Perfecting your blood pressure technique. *Nurs 84* (Canadian ed.) (June) 1984; 14:17.

Quinn A: Thora-Drain III: Closed chest drainage made simpler and safer. *Nurs* (September) 1986; 16:46–51.

Resnick B: Constipation: Common but preventable. *Geriatr Nurs* (July/August) 1985; 6:213–15.

Ritter M: Karaya reconsidered . . . the original skin barrier for persons with an ostomy. *J Enterost Ther* (January/February) 1983; 10:35–36.

Robertson C: Interpreting blood glucose studies. *Nurs 86* (August) 1986; 64.

Shannon ML: Five famous fallacies about pressure sores. *Nurs 84* (October) 1984; 14:34–41.

Shekleton ME, Nield M: Ineffective airway clearance related to artificial airway. *Nurs Clin North Am* (March) 1987; 22:167–78.

Simmons BP: CDC guidelines for prevention of surgical wound infections. *Am J Infect Control* (February) 1983; 11(2):133.

Slahetka F: Dakin's solution for deep ulcers. *Geriatr Nurs* (May/June) 1984; 5:168–69.

Smith DB: Colostomy irrigations—so simple . . . irrigation takes on complex variables and requires individualization in each situation. *J Enterost Ther* (January/February) 1983; 10:22–23.

Sproles KJ: Nursing care of skeletal pins: A closer look. *Orthop Nurs* (January/February) 1985; 4:11–12, 15–19.

Surr CW: Part I: Teaching patients to use the new blood-glucose monitoring products. *Nurs 83* (January) 1983: 42–45.

Surr CW: Part II: Teaching patients to use the new blood-glucose monitoring products. *Nurs 83* (February) 1983: 58–62.

Swearingen PL: *The Addison-Wesley Photo-Atlas of Nursing Procedures.* Addison-Wesley, 1984.

Taylor DL: Wound healing: Physiology, signs, and symptoms. *Nurs 83* (May) 1983; 13(5):44–45.

Todd B: Drugs and the elderly: Topical analgesics. *Geriatr Nurs* (May/June) 1983; 4(3):152, 192, 196.

Todd B: Drugs and the elderly: Using eye drops and ointments safely. *Geriatr Nurs* (January/February) 1983; 4(1):53–56.

Williams P, Bierer B: Wash your hands! *Geriatr Nurs* (March/April) 1984; 5:103–104.

Wimsatt R: Unlocking the mysteries behind the chest wall. *Nurs 85* (November) 1985; 15:58–63.

Wittig P, Semmler-Bertanzi DJ: Pumps and controllers—a nurse's assessment guide. *Am J Nurs* (July) 1983; 83:1022–25.